PRAISE FOR *HEALING WORDS*

Here is a book by a writer whose wisdom, wit, candor, and common sense will inform, enlighten, and entertain any reader. Dr. John Sergent's commentaries, sometimes provocative, often profound, reflect the opinions of a gifted health care professional who, yes, can check your blood pressure and feel your pulse—but also can make you think.

—John Seigenthaler
Chairman Emeritus of the *Tennessean*

I do not know a better doctor and you are not likely to find a better collection of real-life stories written by a doctor than those in this book by John Sergent.

—Lamar Alexander

John Sergent's writing calls us to think deeply about how the important issues in health care connect to the lives and hearts of real people—he encounters us where we live.

—Bob Fisher
President of Belmont University

A powerful compilation of the best that resides in us as human beings. After you have read it, pass it on.

—Wonder Drake, MD
Assistant Professor of Medicine
Vanderbilt University

I always knew John Sergent would amount to something, and sure enough: a healer and a fine writer too.

—Roy Blount Jr.
Author, Humorist

John's columns bring a unique, humorous, personal perspective to current affairs and critical medical issues based upon his deep insights into human nature.

—Hon. Gilbert S. Merritt
U.S. Court of Appeals

You'll laugh, cry, and be filled with wonder at Dr. Sergent's gripping stories of his patients, friends, and family. He is a truly great physician who knows how to listen and heal and inspire young people to live up to his high ideals. These glimpses of his life are so human, so engaging, and so heart-rending that you cannot stop reading. Nashville is fortunate, and medicine is fortunate, to have attracted such a marvelous and balanced intellect—and a marvelous storyteller to boot!
　　　　　—Congressman Jim Cooper

Dr. Sergent is the quintessential mentor: He teaches by what he says, what he does, and by who he is. His book offers wisdom and inspiration and invites us all to re-evaluate what is most important in work and in life.
　　　　　　　—Elisabeth Riviello, MD
　　　　　　　Resident, Internal Medicine
　　　　　　　Brigham and Women's Hospital

John Sergent treats his world in the same way he treats his patients — and we all feel better in the morning. He is a model of civic engagement for us all.
　　　　　　　—Bill Purcell
　　　　　　　Former Mayor, Nashville, Tennessee

Dr. John Sergent's short essays reflect his lively mind and range across a range of medical and human topics with fresh and original insights.
　　　　　　　—Erwin Hargrove
　　　　　　　Professor Emeritus of Political Science
　　　　　　　Vanderbilt University

HEALING
WORDS

A COMPILATION OF THE BEST COLUMNS OF

JOHN SERGENT, MD

Cold Tree Press
Nashville, Tennessee
A Traditional Trade Paperback Press

The columns in this book are reprinted here by permission. Dr. John Sergent's original columns were published by the Nashville Tennessean.

Cold Tree Press is an independent, traditional, trade paperback press committed to introducing fresh, exciting voices to the reading public. It is our mission to take a chance on deserving authors and achieve the highest quality when bringing their words to the marketplace. We believe in the power of words and ideas and strive to introduce readers to new, creative writers.

Published by Cold Tree Press, Nashville, Tennessee. An imprint of Cold Tree Publishing.

For information regarding permission, write to:
Cold Tree Press, 214 Overlook Court, Suite 253, Brentwood, Tennessee 37027.

Library of Congress Number: 2008941112

First Edition: December 2009
10 9 8 7 6 5 4 3 2 1

Cover Photo: Anne Rayner, Vanderbilt University Medical Center

ISBN-13: 978-1-58385-286-6
ISBN-10: 1-58385-286-7

Publisher's Note:

Dr. John Sergent has written a number of columns over the years, starting in 1992. The result of this is a series that shows insight, wisdom, and humor. It is our pleasure to bring a number of the best of these to the readers at large. Regardless of the time frame, the thoughts they present still ring true today. Enjoy!

PREFACE

In 1988 I was named chief of the internal medicine service at St. Thomas Hospital. In addition to the primary duties involving the supervision and education of the Vanderbilt medical students and residents rotating through the hospital, one of my duties involved chairing the hospital's ethics committee. While there are many ethical issues in medicine, most of the issues at St. Thomas in those days involved appropriate care at the end of life. Week after week we dealt with families—and with doctors and nurses—frustrated by the feeling that they had to continue to "do everything," even when hope for meaningful recovery was gone. Probably for the first time I realized the importance of Living Wills, and of having frank, honest discussions with family members regarding your wishes at the end of life.

At that time, the *Tennessean* had an op-ed feature called "The Nashville Eye" and I submitted a few articles on Living Wills. They were published, and, buoyed by the fact that some of them stimulated letters to the editor, which meant that someone had actually read them, I submitted a few more, and began to branch out into areas of health policy and important medical breakthroughs.

One memorable article I owe to the late Sen. Jesse Helms. I don't think I agreed with Sen. Helms on a single issue, but one of his least rational proposals was a bill requiring all health care workers to be tested for HIV every six months and to post the result, similar to the sanitation ratings of restaurants.

The evening after the story on Helms' bill was published in the newspaper, I happened to be at a dinner with Sandra Roberts, then the editorial page editor of the *Tennessean*. I told Sandra the bill was lunacy and said she should write an editorial about it.

"Why don't you?" she replied.

So the next morning I got up early, wrote the column, faxed it to Sandra, and it was published. I was hooked.

During this same period, my longtime friend Dr. Frank Boehm was chair of the ethics committee at Vanderbilt Hospital, and he had written a number of columns as well. One day Frank proposed that we talk to the newspaper about becoming regular columnists. I pretty much laughed it off, but I very much underestimated Frank's chutzpah. A few weeks later we had dinner with Frank Sutherland, the publisher of the paper, and my career as a regular columnist was launched.

The two hundred-plus columns I have written have mostly continued to relate to medical and health policy issues, although at times I couldn't resist writing about personal topics—the marriage of a daughter, the birth of a grandchild, the deaths of dear friends. It is probably because of the personal columns that my best friend and wife of forty-five years, Carole, insisted that we compile some of them into a book. We met with Cold Tree Publishing, they liked the idea, and this book is the result.

—John Sergent, MD

TABLE OF CONTENTS

HEALING WORDS

*A Compilation of the Best Columns of
John Sergent, MD*

I

PATIENTS, STUDENTS,
AND DOCTORS

1

A TALE OF MODERN MEDICINE AND A BOND BETWEEN TWO BROTHERS

And who are the people in this photo?" our guest asked. "I don't recognize either one." He was in our home for the first time, and had been asking about various pictures and pieces of art, no doubt as a way of finding out more about us. "This one we bought after a long, romantic lunch," I said. "And this we bought in a sidewalk cafe. And that was a Father's Day gift." And so on.

When he asked about the photo however, I was speechless. It was a small black-and-white picture in an inconspicuous location, and I had not really looked at it in years. The two young men in the picture are sharing an emotional embrace while standing on a hill overlooking a waterfront. "That's a very old picture," I said. "The one on the left used to be my patient." I tried to move on, but my friend wasn't satisfied. "Tell me more," he insisted.

The young men were brothers. Charley, the older one, was just nineteen when I met him in the summer of 1970. I had returned to Nashville to complete my residency and was working with Dr. John Flexner in hematology. Charley was one of my first patients, and he was dying. Charley had aplastic anemia, the medical term for bone marrow failure. At that point he had been transfused so many times that he had become immune to platelets, and his body would destroy them as soon as they were transfused. He bled constantly, from his gums, his nose, and into his skin, and it was only a matter of time before he would have a fatal hemorrhage, probably into his brain.

One night Dr. Flexner and I had been with Charley for several hours in the emergency room. Charley had a severe headache, probably from bleeding, but there was literally nothing to do. His parents, Elizabeth and the late Dr. Edmund Benz, knew we had nothing to offer in the hospital and decided to take him home, possibly for the last time.

I went home, but too tired to sleep, I picked up a journal that had arrived that day. The lead article told about a new technique of tissue typing to identify people whose platelets match those of their siblings with aplastic anemia. Now too excited to sleep, I waited until dawn and called Elizabeth. We assembled all four of the Benz children by seven-thirty or so, talked to a reference lab in Wisconsin, and sent the samples. By afternoon, our lab thought there was a match, and it was confirmed the next morning. The match was with Charley's brother Yarrott, then a fifteen-year-old, and that afternoon we laboriously removed four units of Yarrott's platelets, a process that took more than three hours in 1970, and that could be done in a few minutes today. We then transfused the platelets into Charley.

I've heard older physicians describe the first time they used penicillin, but what we saw that afternoon was no less dramatic. The oozing from Charley's gums stopped immediately, and when we checked his platelet count, it had gone from near zero to almost a hundred thousand. There were no dry eyes in the room.

Thus began years of twice weekly sessions in the blood bank. Charley and Yarrott developed a bond like no brothers I've known. Yarrott postponed his plans to study design and architecture in order to stay near Charley. And when they did travel, they did it together, always with the assistance of cooperative local medical schools.

Miraculously, after five years, Charley's bone marrow made a complete recovery. Yarrott headed east to pursue his dream, and Charley made up for lost time, fulfilling his lifelong desire to live in the mountains out west. Yarrott turned out to be good at his art, and won a contest to design the exterior of a museum in Philadelphia. Charley went out to visit him, and when he looked at what his brother had created, he was overcome with pride and love, and a friend snapped a photo of their embrace.

But this was not to be a fairy tale. Thirteen years after I first met him and eight years after his remission, Charley developed acute leukemia and died. Yarrott gave the eulogy at his funeral, and the only music was a solo violin playing Beethoven's "Ode to Joy."

That, in part, is the story behind the picture.

2

ANNA

It was a clear, beautiful Sunday afternoon, but as I entered the subway station at 68th and Lexington I was feeling sorry for myself. My two young daughters were growing up fast, and today would have been a nice time to go to the park and ride the carousel or visit the zoo. Or, if they had other plans, the cool, dry air would make the long run around Central Park a real treat for me. However, I had told Anna that I would come to see her, and today was my only opportunity.

I had first met Anna a couple of months earlier, when she came to our arthritis clinic because of widespread pain. She was about seventy but looked older, with wrinkled and waxy skin that was covered with keratoses, the scaly growths so common in the elderly. Several teeth were missing, and the remaining ones were brown and in poor shape. Nevertheless, Anna was bright and witty, and despite her thick German accent, communication was easy. For most of her life she had avoided doctors, and this was her first time to come to Manhattan for medical care. I had hospitalized her, and tests quickly revealed that she had myelodysplastic syndrome, an untreatable disease that inevitably results in death, due either to leukemia or bone marrow failure. Anna had accepted the news calmly, and had made it clear that she wanted to remain at home.

As I banged along on the subway, I wondered what "home" would be like. Anna had told me very little about herself. She had two grown children, but had asked me not to contact them, saying that she would keep them informed about her condition. I knew that she was a widow, that she and her husband had left Germany after the war and had arrived in the United States in the late 1940s, and that was about it, other than details about her disease. However, Anna knew much more about me than I did about her. She was quite curious about my childhood, spent in West Virginia and Kentucky, and about my family. I had told her many details about my wife and children, their ages and where they went to school, and she loved looking at their pictures.

Through a Jewish organization for the elderly, arrangements had been made to bring her to the hospital for transfusions, which she required about every other week. I had found myself calling Anna from time to time just to check on her, and a few days before that Sunday she had seemed unusually anxious to talk. Her pain had increased, but she very much wanted both to remain as lucid as possible, and to minimize the side effects of the drugs. For the first time, she told me that she was scared, not of dying, but of the pain and the unknown. At the end of that conversation I had asked her if she would like me to visit her, and she immediately said yes. We both knew that it was highly unlikely that I could do anything by visiting that I could not do by phone, but I knew the trips to the hospital were painful for her, and I knew how little we had to offer.

So I followed her instructions—Take the Lexington Avenue line downtown and then across to Brooklyn. When I got off the subway, I found myself in a world as different from my childhood as one could imagine. The streets were packed, with outdoor stalls and regular stores doing a booming business. People were bargaining loudly, and several languages were being spoken at once. There were Jews of all varieties, Hassidic Jews with their black hats and earlocks, bearded old rabbis, young boys with yarmulkes, and young families with strollers.

I wandered through this bedlam until I found her building. She lived in a second-floor walk-up, and her apartment had the distinctive look and smell a home acquires when an old person has lived there a long time. The draperies were pulled and it was quiet, a striking contrast to the street below.

As my eyes adjusted to the light, I found myself in a clean, well-cared-for apartment that resembled a 1940s movie set. All the furniture, draperies, pictures, everything, seemed to come from a different time. She sat on the couch and I examined her briefly. Other than some additional weight loss and the persistent bone tenderness, I found nothing remarkable. I told her that we should try another pain medicine to minimize the side effects, and I told her that judging from her skin color, we would need to bring her in again soon for another transfusion.

As I rose to leave, she asked if I would like some orange juice. I said that would be nice, and although she objected briefly, I insisted on getting the juice for the two of us. She told me where the glasses were, and I went into the kitchen.

By the time I returned, she had managed to move herself to a chair by the window, and she said, "Come and sit by me. I have something to show you." In her hands was an old silver picture frame, with a faded three-by-five picture of a young man standing by a white 1930s vintage car. "That is my husband. He owned an ambulance company in Berlin before the war. Isn't he handsome?"

With no trace of bitterness, she told me about him and how much they had loved each other. She didn't tell me anything about the war years; it was as if their lives had not begun until they reached America. She told me of their two children, both of whom were successful and happy, and of the wonderful marriage she had until her husband had died ten years earlier.

She then showed me other pictures—their children and grand-children, some other friends and relatives—but several times came back to the faded picture of her young husband. We talked about many things, and she wanted to know more about my wife and our two daughters, and about where I had grown up. "I've never been to Kentucky," she said. "I hear it's very nice."

When she came for her next transfusion a few days later, it was obvious that the end was near, and that she would not be able to return home. Her white cells and platelets were both near zero, and she was bleeding from her gums. When I told her that

I thought we should call her children, she reluctantly agreed. I assured her that we would not let her suffer, and would try to keep her as lucid as possible.

When her daughter arrived that evening from Montreal, I was surprised by what I saw. She was as beautiful, sophisticated, and "American" as her mother was old, old-fashioned, and European. She was surprised at the deterioration in her mother, and it was obvious that she had not been fully apprised of the seriousness of the illness. Her brother arrived the next morning, and was equally shocked when he saw his mother's terminal state.

Anna died two or three days later. Prior to that, I had had several conversations with the children about their mother, mostly related to medical issues and the importance of adequate pain medications. Her dying was neither the gentlest nor the most painful that I have witnessed, but at the end she was comfortable and her son and daughter were at her side.

A few weeks went by, and then I received a letter from Anna's daughter. "There are some things I think you would want to know about my mother," she wrote. She said that her mother had been raised a Christian, and was a beautiful and sought after girl growing up in Berlin. When she fell in love with, and decided to marry, a Jew, she was the subject of much derision from her friends and relatives, but she was steadfast in her love, and they were married in the early 1930s.

As the Nazis increased their grip on Germany, and Jews began to flee, Anna and her husband felt safe. His business was doing reasonably well, they had established new friends, and besides, they were Germans. Religion was of no particular importance, and by the late thirties their two children were born.

By the time they realized the danger they were in, it was too late. Anna decided that she and her children would be safe, but that her husband was in mortal danger. She announced to all of her friends and anyone else who would listen that he had escaped, leaving her and the children to fend for themselves. For the next six years they lived a secret life, in which he stayed in a hidden crawl space under the floor during the days, and emerged only after darkness. By the end of the war they were all near starvation, since Anna's husband wasn't included in their food ration.

Her daughter's letter went on to say that one of the earliest memories of her childhood was of her mother slapping a Russian officer and being struck in the face by him, which knocked her to the ground and loosened several teeth. The area of Berlin where they lived had been liberated by the Soviets, and after years of living their life in hiding, they were ecstatic that the Nazis were finally defeated. When the Russian officer came into their house, Anna freed her husband from his six years in prison, only to hear the officer make a derogatory comment about "the little Jew." So she had slapped him, and paid for it with several teeth and much pain.

Twenty years have passed since Anna died. I did not continue contact with her daughter, and no longer remember her name. I have had thousands of patients since then, many of whom have their own poignant, heroic stories to tell. But time and again, especially when reading about racist marches in Germany or elsewhere, and the resurgence of anti-Semitism in much of Europe and on U.S. campuses, I think of Anna. She is sitting by the window with the faded three-by-five photo in her lap, remembering another time and place. And I am reminded that, in many cases, physicians receive much more from our patients than we are able to give.

3

TURNING THE TABLES:
A PATIENT HELPS HEAL THE DOCTOR

I admit it. Last Thursday I was deep in self-pity, the disease my father called the mulligrubs. It's a disease that feeds on itself and relishes every bad turn because it allows us to wallow even more in our own misery.

I was getting over the flu, but although the fever was gone and the cough was better, I just didn't feel well. My sleep was still fitful due to coughing and sinus congestion, and my energy level was about half its normal level. I had a busy clinic, made even busier because we had moved some patients when I was acutely ill a few days earlier. Midway through the afternoon I went into an examination room to see Lindsey.

Lindsey is eighteen now, and has been seeing me for juvenile rheumatoid arthritis since she was eleven, when she was referred to me following three weeks of fever, malaise, and arthritis in multiple joints. I still remember that first visit. Lindsey was lovely, a delicate child, small for her age, with big brown eyes that could melt an iceberg. She was in every way a typical eleven-year-old, and all she wanted was to be normal.

Her chart is filled with letters that try to define her limitations in such a way that she could do as many activities as possible—physical education, cheerleading, even attending a regular school as opposed to home schooling. But that was not to be. Lindsey has had a progressive and persistently active disease, and even attending school—much less extracurricular activities—has often been more than she can handle.

Lindsey's mother Debrah works in a factory, but despite lost wages and other job difficulties, she virtually never fails to keep appointments. Knowing Lindsey's difficulties, Debrah tries to maintain an optimistic view, and she and Lindsey talk to each other more like two friends than parent and child. More than once, when I was examining Lindsey's swollen and tender joints, or injecting a joint with cortisone to provide some temporary relief, I looked up and saw big tears rolling down Debrah's cheeks, always wiped away before Lindsey could see them.

Last Thursday was a typical visit. Filled with optimism and promise, we had recently started Lindsey on a new drug, but after two months nothing had changed. Lindsey was in as much pain as ever, and had been so ill on several occasions that she needed help even to get out of bed. She was back in home schooling, far from the dreams she had had for her senior year in high school. I honestly didn't know what else to do.

Lindsey is so young that I have been reluctant to use some of our most aggressive medications, but watching the progression of her disease has made me doubt the wisdom of that approach. Finally, feeling helpless, I put on my best face and tried to persuade Lindsey and Debrah that it was too soon to change medicines, and that we would reevaluate her in two months.

Lindsey and her mother left, and I continued seeing my patients. Half an hour later, as I was coming out of an examination room, there stood Lindsey and Debrah, and before I could say anything, Lindsey handed me a beautiful pink rose. "You seemed down today," she said, "and we just wanted to cheer you up." I was speechless. We hugged, and then they smiled and walked away, Lindsey limping and leaning on her mother.

And I went back into a room to see the next patient.

4

THE DOCTOR AS PATIENT

I was jogging along West End Avenue when a friend blew his horn as he passed by. As I waved, I misjudged the curb, landed hard, and felt a sharp pain in my pelvis. Over the next two days I was a little sore, and I also felt fatigued and lost my appetite. I tried to go ahead with a planned family vacation, but after two days of increasing symptoms, we flew home and I went straight to bed.

Lying in bed, I tried to figure out what could be wrong. The pain from the injury had become so severe that I assumed I must have fractured a bone. But why should I feel so bad? Feeling around in the tender area in my pelvis, I found a small lymph node that was a little tender. At about that time I had the first of several hard, bed-shaking chills, and was taken to the hospital. Although I had been in robust health only a few days earlier, the bone pain, the lymph node, and now the chills made the diagnosis obvious to me: leukemia or a lymphatic malignancy.

The next day or two are a blur, but I had several more chills followed by bed-soaking sweats, underwent numerous diagnostic tests, and then miraculously I began to feel better. I had developed an unusual but very treatable infection at the site of an injury caused by muscle tearing away from bone. I was in the hospital for eight days, and was back to work part-time a couple of weeks later.

Dr. Franz Ingelfinger, the late editor of the *New England Journal of Medicine*, wrote of his experience as a patient with cancer of the esophagus. Being ill had affected him so profoundly that he suggested, only partially tongue-in-cheek, that no one who had not sustained a serious illness be accepted to medical school. I know now what Dr. Ingelfinger meant, because my illness, while totally cured, changed the way I approach the practice of medicine.

In the first place, I realize how much anxiety surrounds illness, especially if there are undiagnosed symptoms. If I, a specialist in rheumatology and internal medicine, had concluded I must have a malignancy, how can I downplay the fear and anxiety other people may feel? I learned also that it is very helpful to tell people what they *don't* have (cancer, for example), even while trying to make a correct diagnosis. Further, I learned that diagnostic tests can be a miserable experience. Trying to lie still on a cold, hard x-ray table for an hour or so is difficult under the best of circumstances, but when in pain it can be torture.

I have also come to appreciate much of the complaining I had largely ignored in the past. It is very difficult for a patient to understand a particular diagnostic report when miserably constipated, and the daily barrage of blood drawing and intravenous medications can make the condition of one's veins the most important fact of daily existence.

More than ever before, I appreciate the value of kindness and gentleness on the part of physicians and nurses. There are even those who believe that these attributes actually speed physical healing. I'm not sure about that, but I know that illness is stressful enough at best, and that friendly, compassionate physicians and nurses can reduce a patient's pain and anxiety a great deal.

While we certainly won't go so far as to require a major prior illness of all of our medical school applicants, Dr. Ingelfinger was right. It would change the practice of medicine for the better.

5

SHEDDING CULTURAL PREJUDICES
IS THE BEST MEDICINE

On the afternoon of September 11, 2001, after I was satisfied that my family and friends in New York were okay, I sent an e-mail to Yasmine Ali, a former student, to let her know that her friends in Nashville were thinking of her.

She is a Muslim, but the subject had come up only tangentially in our first meetings. Except for the Palestinian flag lapel pin she proudly wore in honor of the homeland of one of her parents, nothing about her seemed anything other than American. Her skin was a little darker than some of her classmates, but her speech, her gait, her mannerisms—everything—were as American as they come. The daughter of physicians, she was one of those students who seem to inhale medicine. She loved learning and it was obvious that she could not get enough of it.

My main contact with Yasmine had come rather early, in her third year of medical school. Then, a few months later, she asked to meet with me. I assumed it was to discuss possible residency programs, although that discussion usually doesn't take place until later. When she walked into my office, I knew the subject was not about residencies. Gone was the easy-going, happy student I had known. Something was up, and it was very serious.

Teary-eyed, she said she was going to get a C in a major course, and she knew that grade, while technically passing, would doom her chances of getting into a competitive residency program. She was distraught. She told me that a resident had made what she took to be anti-Muslim comments about some of their patients, and she didn't know how to deal with it. So what she did, as is understandable, was to withdraw and avoid contact with that resident as much as possible.

Unfortunately, much of the grade of third-year medical students depends on their active involvement in the care of their patients. Part student, part young doctor-to-be, they are expected to do their share of the work of obtaining histories, doing examinations, and, most importantly, going to the literature and bringing new knowledge to the care of their patients. We discussed better ways of dealing with these issues if they came up in the future, and I discussed the matter with the department chair.

I am glad to report that the story ended happily. Thanks to an extremely good grade on her exam, she did not receive a C, and she is now happily in the second year of an excellent residency program, where she was chosen last year as the outstanding member of the house staff.

Incidentally, her response to my e-mail of 9/11 was just what I would have predicted. She had already organized Muslim students at her new university, to teach people about what Islam really means, and about the peace and tolerance that are at its roots.

When the war in Iraq began, I realized I hadn't heard from Yasmine in several months, so I e-mailed her again just to check in. She responded immediately, and told me the following story. One of her patients that day was a farmer who was wearing American flag suspenders. As he was leaving, he turned around and asked, "Where are you from originally?"

When Yasmine heard the word "originally," she thought, "Oh, God, here it comes." "Tennessee," she replied, "but my parents are from the Middle East."

"I thought so," he said. "I just want you to know that when I watched TV last night I had tears in my eyes. There are twelve-year-old children over there losing their fathers. I don't know why I'm telling you this, us bein' strangers and all, but somehow I feel better now. I just wanted you to know."

We are a wonderfully heterogeneous country, but we are at a major turning point. As my friend John Compton, emeritus professor of philosophy at Vanderbilt, pointed out recently, we readily explain away excesses of Christianity, like the Crusades, the Inquisition, Northern Ireland, and Christianity's role in the Holocaust, yet we paint Islam with a single brush, quick to stereotype members of the world's second largest religion.

Pre-judging and casting people in ethnic or demographic roles is always dangerous, whether they are Muslims born in Tennessee or farmers wearing American flag suspenders. God Bless America. All of us.

6

RESIDENT PHYSICIANS
LEARN TO HELP EACH OTHER

About six weeks into my first year of residency, usually called the internship, I hit the wall. We were on call six nights a week, and I had gone through a week in which all of my patients came into the hospital at night. Sleep had been erratic and often interrupted, and on Saturday night I had none at all.

Before leaving around noon on Sunday, we had chart rounds in which the two interns and two residents who worked together reviewed all the patients, so that the team remaining on call would be familiar with all the problems. One of the residents later became a good friend of mine, but that Sunday morning he could do nothing but criticize. Every single patient of mine, according to him, needed additional work, and needed it that day. It meant some lab work here, a follow-up procedure there, a review of medical records somewhere else, all in all, several hours of effort, especially at the inefficient pace of a new intern. The other resident on our team, Jay Jensen, had said little during chart rounds, but when we finished he pulled me aside and said, "All of this can wait a while. Go home and get some sleep."

I called Carole and told her to cancel our plans for the afternoon, and I tried to get some of the work done, but my brain literally had shut down. After a hopelessly inefficient hour in which lines on the page ran together in a blur, I decided to take Jay's advice, and I went across the street to our apartment. Quite unexpectedly, as I walked into the building I found myself crying. "I'm not cut out for this," I told Carole. She told me to get some sleep, and when I awoke a few hours later I felt a little better. We ate dinner, and I went back to the hospital for what I expected to be a long night of catching up.

I pulled the first chart from the rack, and there, in Jay's bold handwriting, was a note describing the required procedure; it was signed, "Jensen." On and on it went. Every single chart, none of which belonged to any of Jay's patients, was complete and up-to-date. Jay had given up his free afternoon to bail me out. Best of all, on the shelf where I kept my equipment, he had left a clipboard with all my patients organized according to what needed to be done, and when. I adopted his system and for the rest of the year I never again fell behind.

The years of training after medical school are called "residencies," a throwback to the days when the doctors actually lived in the hospital. It is a strange time of being part student and part hospital employee, and still today the hours are long and the pay is low. Increasingly, over the past few years, there has been a growing realization that fatigue has a major impact on performance. In addition, the public has a strong vested interest in seeing that people in critical positions like airplane pilots, doctors and others, get adequate periods of rest. So, beginning this July, medical residents in the United States will be limited to eighty hours on call per week. That's not a misprint. They're still working very hard.

I haven't seen Jay Jensen since 1967, but I wrote him in the mid-'80s to thank him once again for bailing me out that Sunday afternoon. A couple of weeks later his reply came. I should have expected it. "I remember that month and what a great time we had, John. But I don't remember that Sunday. Great to hear from you, though."

To Jay, you see, helping people in trouble was just part of the job.

7

WONDER

Except for her unusual first name, Wonder Puryear, who graduated from Vanderbilt last month, is in almost every way a typical brand new physician. Along with most of her classmates, she is busy packing up and preparing to move to another city to embark on a new phase of her young life. Wonder is headed to Baltimore and an internship at Johns Hopkins.

Like many of her classmates, Wonder did some research in medical school and she is excited by the phenomenon of scientific discovery. Again like her classmates, Wonder loves clinical medicine with its challenges and rewards. She thinks she would like a career in academic medicine where she could combine research and teaching with patient care. As many as half of her classmates plan similar careers at this stage in their lives.

There is a great deal of self-selection involved in going to medical school, so it comes as no surprise that medical students like Wonder bond very closely with their patients, and medical schools are full of stories of patients who refuse to undergo a procedure or operation until they have a chance to confer with their "doctor," the medical student assigned to their case.

During her third year internal medicine rotation, Wonder was required to discuss a case with a small group of students. The patient was an elderly Middle Tennessee farm woman with advanced emphysema. As we entered her room, she appeared to be uncomfortable, and she was obviously in the midst of complaining to her husband about something. Just then she looked up, her eyes brightened, and she held out her arms to Wonder and said to her husband, "It's all right, Honey. My doctor is here."

So there it was, a very ordinary event involving this very typical medical student and her patient, but for one thing: Wonder is black, and her patient is white.

For those of us who grew up in the segregated South, and who remember when the wards at Vanderbilt Hospital were still segregated (as they were at Johns Hopkins, incidentally), there was a sense of awe, indeed wonder, at what had occurred. Here was this young Southern black woman, whose mother had supported her family by working in a factory after Wonder's father died when she was eight, and here was this elderly, rural white woman, who had probably never before had a woman, much less a black woman, as a doctor.

Yet with no fanfare, and probably without even thinking about it very much, these two individuals had bridged a chasm of mistrust and intolerance that would have seemed impossible only a few years ago. Wonder was the doctor, and she cared deeply about her patient, even if the best she had to offer was a comforting smile. Her patient saw this, and somehow recognized that aspect as what was really important about Wonder, not her gender or the color of her skin.

The statistics are still abysmal, of course. Blacks still trail the rest of the country in income, educational level, and many other areas, including proportionate representation in medicine. We still have a long way to go. But amidst the Nation of Islam, skinheads, black separatists, the Klan, and all the rest, we should not forget to take pride in what progress has been made.

This progress can be told by statistics that reveal increasing involvement by blacks in politics, business, and the professions. But it can best be portrayed by individual stories, like that of people like Wonder Puryear, who go about living ordinary lives and in so doing, they turn what is ordinary into the remarkable.

8

LADYDOC

When I entered medical school thirty-one years ago, our class of fifty-two included two women. Actually, we called them girls in those days, but we usually called ourselves boys as well, and the term "politically correct" had not yet made it into the lexicon.

At any rate, the two women, both very bright, must have felt pretty lonely. There was only one woman in the class ahead of us, and I can only recall three women on the faculty, one in anatomy and two in pediatrics. There were very few women residents as well.

Medical school turned out to be rough for both of the women in my class, which in retrospect is not surprising, given the times. They each married classmates and were subsequently divorced. One of them dropped out for a year and graduated a year late.

This week a new class begins medical school at Vanderbilt. Of 104 entering first-year students, forty-five are women. On their first day of school they will be greeted by a woman dean of students, and the house staff and faculty are liberally stocked with women, though as yet there are few women departmental chairs in any U.S. medical school and only one so far at Vanderbilt.

With such striking demographic change over these thirty-one years, one cannot help but pause and reflect on the impact of this transformation. Have we simply increased the pool of applicants, or have women brought about a basic change in medicine?

The answer is elusive, though some changes are obvious. For example, we have learned to be flexible in our residency programs to allow for pregnancy and motherhood, and we have learned that women are much less willing to see a future devoted entirely to medicine at the expense of family and other concerns. It has been twenty years since I heard the phrase, "Medicine is a jealous mistress."

In objective measurements of quality of care delivered, women perform at least as well as men. Indeed, a study in a recent issue of the *New England Journal of Medicine* indicated that women are more likely to have routine Pap smears and mammograms if their physicians are women. This difference was especially marked among younger physicians, implying that young male physicians may not be as comfortable dealing with these matters as they should be.

But the important changes brought about by women are much more subjective. Women physicians more often seem to form collegial relationships with nurses, social workers, and others, and to see themselves as part of a team of caregivers rather than autonomous decision-makers. More importantly, they are often willing to discuss their own feelings and emotions, and to allow them to show on occasion.

Ultimately, women have forced all of us in medicine to re-examine our profession and our professional lives. If it is acceptable for women physicians to take time off for dance recitals and soccer games, then it is unacceptable for their male counterparts not to do the same. If women physicians sometimes cry as they sit by the bedside of a terminally ill patient, then maybe we will create an outlet for men who feel equally angry and frustrated by the suffering of our patients, yet have had to maintain a stoic, "masculine" image.

I once asked a male surgeon about a young female surgeon, and he paid her his highest compliment by saying, "She operates like a man."

Maybe the time will come when the highest compliment for a male physician will be, "He cares for his patients like a woman."

9

WITH NEW DOCTORS LIKE DANA, MEDICINE IS IN GOOD HANDS

The number of medical school applicants nationally has been falling steadily. Some doctors are retiring early, and others are leaving the practice of medicine and entering the business world. The legal and financial woes of medical groups routinely appear in the pages of the *Wall Street Journal*. Woe is us...maybe...maybe not.

The fact is, medicine is undergoing a fundamental restructuring, much as the auto industry, communications, computer manufacturing, and many other segments of the economy have done in the past couple of decades. When you are in the middle of such a process it is painful, especially for those of us who are old enough to have developed set ways of doing things. But we aren't the future of medicine. The future is those young men and women who are today's medical students.

I have the good fortune of interacting on a regular basis with medical students and because of them, I don't share the doom and gloom I hear from others. I want to tell you about just one. Her name is Dana Deaton.

Dana is from Nashville, and is a 1999 graduate of Princeton. While there, she got involved with something called Princeton Project 55, a program started by alumni of the university's class of 1955. It has undertaken many useful endeavors, including placement of Princeton students in summer jobs at a variety of non-profit organizations around the country. Dana got involved with a project inspired by Dr. Gordon Douglas, an infectious diseases expert and member of the Princeton Class of '55, who is the former chairman of internal medicine at Cornell and a former executive at Merck. His goal was quite straightforward: to solve the world's growing problem of tuberculosis. When Dana graduated, she went to work for the Project 55 Tuberculosis Initiative.

It sounds ridiculously naïve. How can a brand new college graduate do anything about the world's second largest infectious cause of death? More to the point, how can she, or anyone for that matter, effect great change when the biggest beneficiaries of controlling TB are third world countries that can't pay for it? What she and her colleagues did, and what others continue to do, however, was simply keep their eyes on the ball. She educated members of Congress. She worked with people at the Centers for Disease Control. She worked with the World Health Organization. She wrote letters to the editor of *The New York Times* and other newspapers.

And here's what has happened. The Project 55 Tuberculosis Initiative received a grant for $100 thousand from an affiliate of the Gates Foundation to increase public awareness of TB. U.S. funding for worldwide TB treatment went from practically nothing to $35 million in 2000, and to $60 million in 2001. They have worked to get the Centers for Disease Control TB budget doubled to $280 million. Thanks in part to their efforts, TB research sponsored by the National Institutes of Health has increased from less than $2 million to $80 million in ten years. They have worked with the Rockefeller Foundation to develop the Global Alliance for TB Drug Development, and two major drug and vaccine proposals are under way. The list goes on and on.

Dr. Douglas had told me about Dana, and I looked her up right before the holidays. She is a petite blonde who looks even younger than her years, and whose enthusiasm is so great that she literally never stops smiling. As we concluded our meeting, which left me smiling as much as she was, I asked her what she was going to do over the holidays. I assumed she would give herself a well-deserved rest after her first semester in medical school. "I'm going to work on my job for next summer," she said. "I want to go to

Africa and work in a clinic, to see firsthand some of the problems I worked on."

I just happened to get to know Dana through my friendship with Dr. Douglas, but the really great news is that she's not atypical at all. Medical schools are full of people with similar interests, enthusiasm, and idealism. And that keeps me from listening to the preachers of doom and gloom.

10

THE CARING QUOTIENT

At Vanderbilt, as at nearly all U.S. medical schools, the third year is the beginning of clinical medicine. After two years of study of the basic sciences of medicine, the students are finally allowed to be part of a clinical team.

Dr. Roger des Prez, chief of medicine at Nashville Veterans Administration Hospital, and professor of medicine at Vanderbilt, has suggested that we should have some sort of ceremony as students enter their third year, to emphasize that for the rest of their lives, the purpose of their education is to improve the care of their patients. As he puts it, "Education is self-centered from kindergarten until the third year of medical school. From then on, all meaningful education focuses on the care of the patient."

"Amy" was a typical third-year student. During her five weeks on my service, she was assigned to an intern-resident team, and she took histories and performed physical examinations on two or three new patients each week. I read her write-ups carefully, as did the younger doctors working with her, and we all complimented her on her strengths and worked with her on her weaknesses. For all of her patients, she was expected to participate in any procedures and be knowledgeable about their illnesses and their medications.

Because the education is patient-centered, it is difficult and always subjective to grade third-year students, but after five weeks I felt that I knew Amy quite well. Her written work had shown steady improvement, her fund of knowledge was increasing with each patient, and she was conscientious and diligent in performing her share of the work involved in the care of her patients. After reviewing all of this and considering her bedside manner and degree of comfort around her patients, I felt that she deserved a solid average grade, but I secretly hoped she would do extremely well on the final exam and pull herself up into the top part of her class.

But grades don't tell the whole story. Several weeks after Amy went on to further rotations, a brief letter appeared on my desk from a recent patient who had responded to a routine questionnaire. After checking the appropriate boxes regarding food, the X-ray department, and so on, she had attached a handwritten note. She wrote that she had been admitted to the hospital for experimental chemotherapy, but after admission her cancer was discovered to be too far advanced. Her physician had told her that further therapy would only make her remaining time more miserable. She said she was crushed, her last hope for a prolonged remission now gone.

She went on to say that her doctor and the nurses were very caring, but that she could not have endured the night if it were not for the attention, love, and compassion of her medical student. Amy had stayed with her and cried with her after she had received the news, and had returned several times during the night to check on her. As the patient was leaving the next morning, Amy was there with a goodbye hug.

I don't know what specialty Amy will select, where she will settle, or whether she will go into research or clinical practice. I don't even know if she did well or poorly on the examination. I do know, however, that all the college and medical school and exam scores couldn't tell me as much about what kind of doctor Amy will become as that one brief letter from her patient.

11

THE SEASON BRINGS A CONSTANT
SEARCH FOR HAPPY ENDINGS

The other day I talked to a medical student who has decided to go into geriatrics. She is as bright and engaging as anyone you'll ever meet. When I asked her how she arrived at her decision, she told me about Mr. H, a man she had helped care for in the hospital. He had terminal throat cancer and could only talk by writing. Difficult as it was, she came to know Mr. H well, admiring the fact that he maintained his sense of humor despite his condition.

After his discharge she continued to visit him periodically, driving sixty miles each way to an extended care facility in his hometown. She learned that Mr. H had lived a rough life and had many regrets, mostly because of broken relationships. She then told me that he died a couple of weeks ago.

"Had he healed any of his relationships?" I asked.

"No. He died alone," she replied, "except for me."

As I drove home that night, the weather had turned sharply colder. My car was just beginning to warm up as I cut through the park near my home. I was thinking of Mr. H and his medical student when I suddenly saw the little sub-compact car I'd been noticing for months. Its owner is a woman who appears to be in her forties, and who spends most of her time sitting in her car. Occasionally the car is gone for a few hours, but it always returns, backed into the same parking space. I've seen her outside the car only two or three mornings, when she was doing some unusual flapping exercises with her arms, and then she walked around the park. Every other time

I've seen her she has been sitting alone in the car, seemingly intent on something she constantly fools with in her lap. She never looks up as I walk or drive by. I've seen her there in all kinds of weather, and at all times of the day and night.

One time I pulled in beside her, and sat there for at least a minute. Her window was rolled up but the slight turn of her head told me she was aware of my presence. She didn't look up. Finally realizing we were not going to establish eye contact, I said, "Are you okay?" Without actually looking at me, hands busy in her lap, she nodded yes. "Do you need anything? Can I do anything for you?" I practically shouted. She shook her head no and waved her hand as if to dismiss me. That was a few weeks ago.

The night I heard about Mr. H was by far the coldest of the season, and I slowed down as I passed the little car. I could barely see the top of the woman's head resting against the window. She was covered with a blanket and appeared to be sleeping. I didn't stop. I rationalized that if I was too persistent, I might run her away from a place that must feel safe to her, and that whatever I did, the story was not likely to have a happy ending.

Christmas and other holidays are wonderful times for those of us with friends and families. They are times to strengthen relationships, relive family history, and just enjoy one another's company. For the lonely, however, Christmas can be a painful reminder of what is missing. As a patient once told me, "Christmas is the longest day of the year. Sometimes I don't even want to get out of bed." I then remembered the stories of her estranged brother, her chronically depressed mother, and her own fractured relationships. It's little wonder that depression, alcohol abuse, and suicide all increase at this time of the year.

Reaching out to people has its risks. First, your efforts may not be wanted, and you may be rebuffed. Then again, you know that no matter what you do, things may not get any better. Nevertheless, the medical student took a risk: though she knew in advance that Mr. H's story would not end happily, she was able to comfort a dying man in his last days. And she probably changed her own life in the process.

This morning, I had determined I was going to stop and try once more to talk to the woman in the car. When I got to the park, she wasn't there.

12

BETH

There is a lot to learn in medical school...genetics, immunology, clinical skills, you name it. Medical school is four years crammed with about as much as we can throw at the students. There is one thing, though, that must be learned but can't be taught. It is critical that our students learn about their patients; it is just as critical that they learn about themselves. Beth, who prefers to keep her last name anonymous, is a rising fourth-year student at Vanderbilt who learned a lot about herself from an interaction with one particular patient, Bill Weaver. This is Beth's story in her own words:

"I have Hepatitis C." Much to my dismay, this was not a patient's response to my history taking, but rather my husband's report of his own lab result. A surgery resident, he had been cut during an emergency operation several weeks earlier and was now infected with Hepatitis C. Two days before this, we had learned that I was pregnant. While the news of my husband's infection was jolting, we were buoyed by the joy of anticipating our first child. One bad thing, one good—a balance. But then a week later the bleeding started, and our child was gone.

*I was devastated. I am a person of faith, but my faith was shaken and my anger aroused. How could this happen to **me**? I am a medical student, not a patient or a patient's wife. My own patients became my dreaded work, the barriers to my being able to leave the hospital to grieve a little more.*

Then I met Mr. Weaver. Our teacher had told us that he had multiple sclerosis and that despite his illness he had worked tirelessly to help others, often calling on his friends, many of whom are in positions of prominence, for various projects aimed primarily at inner-city youth.

We walked into the room. Mr. Weaver appeared to be in his sixties. He had a tracheotomy tube and a feeding tube in place. He was unable to use any of his four limbs. He was propped in bed, smiling. His speech was slurred and difficult to understand. He proudly pointed out the picture of his grandchildren on the bedside table and joked with us about his friend, our teacher.

As we left the room, it was all I could do not to burst into tears. I was overwhelmed by two realizations. First, though some bad things had happened to me, some much worse things had happened to Mr. Weaver. He had chosen to live his life fully nonetheless. He had chosen joy and generosity and perseverance. I had chosen self-pity. None of us is immune to the hardships of life. What matters is not so much which hardships we endure, but rather how we choose to respond. In meeting Mr. Weaver I was "kicked in the pants." I was inspired, and I found some hope.

*Second, it occurred to me that when Mr. Weaver was diagnosed, it was really awful. Just as I felt that my husband's diagnosis and our miscarriage "should not have happened" to us, Mr. Weaver must have felt likewise. Disease is painful. It robs us of physical and mental capacities; it robs us of hopes and dreams. I have a good friend whose husband died in his early seventies. She said, "Just because you get older doesn't mean it makes **sense** that the people you love get sick and die. You don't get used to it." Just as I had felt that my own suffering didn't make sense, **all** of my patients will feel the same way at some level. I had gotten so caught up in being a "good medical student" in the last year that I had forgotten what I used to know: being a good physician includes sharing in our patient's suffering.*

As teachers we concentrate on the written curriculum, but know that equally important is the unwritten or hidden curriculum. The unwritten curriculum is what we teach by our attitudes and our values. Beth reminds us that for medical students there is yet a third curriculum, that which we learn from our patients. Meeting Bill Weaver at a critical point in her own life allowed Beth to gain invaluable insight into herself. Her patients will forever benefit.

13

DR. TOM BRITTINGHAM

In a profession famous for its poor penmanship, Dr. Tom Brittingham's was among the worst and was certainly the most recognizable. As we presented our patients to him, TEB, as he was called by all his students, stood at the blackboard and laboriously took notes, oblivious to the fact that we could read scarcely a word he wrote.

His notes on our reports were largely for himself, because we soon found that no matter how well we prepared, TEB always knew our patients better than we did. For anemic patients he made his own blood smear, and usually discovered some previously unnoticed abnormality. Or if there were features missing from a previous illness, he found some obscure relative or medical records librarian who provided the missing information.

Because he apparently recognized the limitations of his penmanship, TEB typed most of his chart notes. Amazingly, his ancient black Smith Corona left a record as recognizably TEB as did his handwriting. Rare was the intern who did not get a sudden chill upon opening a patient's chart early in the morning to discover a typed note with the top-half of the "e" solid black, the "t" a little above the line, and all capital letters with just a trace of red at the bottom. The note inevitably raised some previously omitted diagnostic point or attached critical importance to an overlooked piece of laboratory data.

As familiar as his handwriting was, so too was his peeling, ancient white Thunderbird with the driver's side door that opened only sporadically and with a mind of its own. Puttering along between Vanderbilt Hospital and his beloved patients in the Nashville General Hospital clinic, the "Brittingham-mobile" was like an old horse, reliably going back and forth to the same parking spaces despite its appearance of impending collapse.

It was at General Hospital that TEB first showed many of us what being a doctor was all about. He had been in Nashville only a few months, and we were still learning his ways. It was Christmas time, and faculty members were covering all of the hospital units and emergency rooms so the interns and residents could have a party. TEB had asked for the Nashville General emergency room. He showed up dressed in his usual shirt and tie with no jacket, and the intern went off to the party.

The next morning when the intern came to relieve him, TEB was not a pretty sight. Sleepless and unshaven, he was splattered with blood, vomit, and assorted other fluids. Over the intern's objections, however, he refused to leave until he had finished taking care of all his patients. It was a cold, rainy Christmas Eve morning, and after TEB left, the intern breathed a sigh of relief. As is often the case on such days, the emergency room was not very busy.

Then a couple of hours later, a strange thing happened. A patient showed up with one of TEB's barely legible notes. A second soon followed, then another, and another. "His left lung sounds worse; he needs a chest X-ray," one note said. "His pain is no better. He probably needs admission," went another. And so it went into the evening, as the old white Thunderbird made its rounds of house calls on TEB's patients from the night before.

Despite his leaving Vanderbilt in 1980 and his subsequent death in 1986, whenever any of his former students and residents get together and discuss the people who really made a difference in their lives, the conversation always begins, "Do you remember the time TEB…"

14

A HEALING ART

The parents jump to their feet as the doctor enters the room, startled by this intrusion into the quiet of their son's sleep. Despite the morning's conversation in which they were told that the doctor would return that evening to go over the test results, the sudden realization that the moment has arrived is filled with tension. The looks on their faces plead, "Please tell us it's all a mistake, that he really isn't that sick. Please give us some good news." But the news isn't good. The disease is aggressive and without therapy will cause permanent disability or death.

All afternoon, as the reports kept coming in, the doctor could not get this family off his mind. The son, the picture of health only a few weeks before, is now barely able to get out of bed. All of the family's problems—business, financial, the older sister who has decided to drop out of college—suddenly are minuscule compared to the magnitude of the decisions to be made now.

"How do I tell them?" the doctor wonders. Trying to put himself in their place, he knows he would want the truth. Gone are the days when doctors skirted around bad diagnoses, like cancer, by using buzzwords such as "growth" or "tumor." The truth may be brutal, but the doctor wants this family to know the positive side as well, that with good treatment and luck, the sick young man lying in bed could be restored to good health.

The treatment options all have potentially serious side effects, and the doctor knows that perseverance will be required and that the patient must be confident that it's all worth it. So the doctor delivers the bad news using all the positives he can muster: youth, early diagnosis, and the absence of irreversible changes. Then, there are the treatment options themselves. Before 1960 or thereabouts, the doctor would simply have prescribed the treatment deemed best. But under the doctrine of informed consent, and with our medically savvy population, today's physicians discuss all the reasonable treatment options, including their relative risks and benefits.

Then what? In this new world of shared medical decision-making, is that the role of the doctor? Does his or her job end when all the options are described, or does the physician have an additional responsibility, that of making a specific recommendation?

Dr. Franz Ingelfinger, himself dying of cancer at the time, delivered a famous lecture in the 1980s at Harvard Medical School, in which he said that for a physician just to lay out the options and tell the patient to choose is tantamount to medical malpractice. To do that deprives the patient of the one thing that the physician is ideally equipped to give: medical judgment as it applies to a specific patient. The fact is, of course, that a computer could describe the treatment options, probably more accurately than the physician, but a computer can't consider the intangible variables: the intelligence and reliability of this family, the toughness and ambition of this young man, and the already strong relationship the doctor has forged with them.

And a computer can't look the patient in the eye, touch his arm, and tell him it is all right to cry, and then say, "So those are your options. And despite the risks and uncertainties, I believe the best treatment for you is…"

15

DR. JOHN JOHNSON

Do you ever have days when, in the middle of chaos, something wonderful comes out of nowhere to put things in perspective? Last Tuesday was such a day for me.

For a variety of reasons, things were not going very well; I was feeling harried and hopelessly behind. The graduating medical students had invited me to a luncheon to thank the faculty, and I really didn't have time for it. However, since many of the students I had known and taught were scattering all over the country, I felt I had to go, despite being worried about how late I would have to work to make up for the time at the luncheon.

As I walked in, however, I realized this was no ordinary good-bye luncheon. Seated at the main table, surrounded by his family, was Dr. John Johnson, a friend and colleague for the past thirty-five years. The students had decided to honor Dr. Johnson, who is professor of medicine at Vanderbilt and chief of the medical service at St. Thomas Hospital. Dr. Johnson suffers from a progressive neurological disorder similar to amyotrophic lateral sclerosis (Lou Gehrig's disease), and the disease has progressed to the point that he reluctantly must retire from teaching. In his honor, the students created an annual award to be given to a faculty member who is especially focused on the needs of students.

John has an extraordinary intellect. In rheumatology circles, his familiarity with complex immunology and his ability to teach those concepts, are the stuff of legend. However, it was apparent from the comments of many students that they chose to honor him not for his intellect, but for his humanity.

One after the other, comments carried the same refrain: in Dr. Johnson, they know they have a professor who loves them and cares about them. Despite more than a few teary eyes, John thanked the students and, one by one, his family members, beginning with his father, the late Dr. Hollis Johnson. John's speech was slowed by his illness, but he was never more persuasive. The love he feels for his family, his colleagues, and his students was palpable to everyone in attendance.

None of us can know how we would deal with a progressive, incurable disease until it actually happens to us. Some never get past the stage of denial, making it impossible for loved ones to be honest in their conversations. Others get trapped in anger and spend their time in self pity, always asking, "Why me?" Still others choose exotic, unproven therapies, wasting time and money, and again making it difficult for people to be honest with the afflicted loved one.

John Johnson has chosen to look his disease squarely in the eye. Although he was willing to try an experimental form of therapy, he has been honest with himself and others as his disease has progressed. Despite the seriousness of his condition, he has also maintained his sense of humor, for instance, commenting recently that his wife, Ellen, complained that his slowed speech made it sound like she was taking dictation from him.

As I looked around the room at the red-eyed students, it was apparent that they would take much of John Johnson with them as they begin their residency education. They will remember his lectures on immunology and rheumatology, and they will remember the high ideals he carried with him into his clinical practice. Most of all, though, they will remember the honesty and courage with which he has faced his illness. And I'll carry with me the memory of the busy day when I had the good fortune to share in something beautiful.

As another favorite teacher, Dr. John Tarpley, pointed out in his parting remarks to the students, when our careers approach their end, the important ledger is not financial. It is the measure of our interpersonal relationships and the impact we've had on others. By that accounting, John Johnson has accumulated a fortune.

16

WITHOUT ENGLISH,
SHE NEEDS MORE THAN MEDICINE

When I first met "Maria," as I'll call her, she was lying on her back, motionless except for her eyes, which darted back and forth among the team of doctors and medical students now responsible for her care. The look on her face was one of sheer terror. We tried to comfort her, but she only stared at us and did not respond. Sitting quietly in the corner were her wrinkled, leather-skinned mother along with her sister and brother.

Maria and her family did not speak English. She was a so-called "illegal alien," a member of the predominantly Mexican workforce responsible for construction, landscaping, and agricultural jobs all over America. Although Maria had been in this country for four years, she lived and worked in an entirely Spanish-speaking community where learning English is not only unnecessary, it is practically useless. Her mother and siblings had recently arrived in Nashville on emergency visas.

Maria was desperately ill when she showed up at our emergency room. As is often the case when people have no health insurance, and doubly so for undocumented aliens, she had put off seeking medical care as long as possible. She soon developed respiratory failure and spent nearly a week on a ventilator in the intensive care unit.

A condition known as ICU psychosis is a mixture of depression, delirium, and frank psychosis, and is sometimes seen after intensive care unit stays of more than a few days. People affected are often paranoid and delusional. Many factors are responsible for the condition including toxicity from the illness itself, sleep deprivation, and the loss of normal sensory input. In Maria's case, in which she did not understand most of her caregivers, the ICU experience must have been an unimaginable horror.

When we met her, Maria's physical condition had improved enough for her to be removed from the ventilator and transferred to a regular room, but she was still extremely ill. Her limbs were bloated and weak, she was jaundiced, her blood counts were critically low, and she had severe kidney disease. We were able to establish a diagnosis and begin therapy, but we knew that her physical condition was only part of our challenge. Equally daunting were the communication and social issues involved in her care.

With a Spanish vocabulary largely limited to words like *cerveza* (beer) and *baño* (bathroom), I was totally dependent on Maria's intern and medical student, both of whom spoke Spanish. Day after day, I watched them gently explain to Maria and her family what was happening. My inability to understand their words allowed me to focus on the non-verbal communication that was taking place, and I saw the impact of a warm tone of voice, a caring smile, and, most of all, a gentle touch. Almost miraculously, Maria's medical problems slowly improved; at the same time, she began to climb out of her shell. At first it consisted only of cooperating with our examinations. Gradually she started to nod in answer to questions by the student and intern, and eventually she began to say a few words.

After several days in our care, we finally saw her smile. We had asked her ever-present family to try to get her into a chair, and when we walked in, there she was—upright, hair combed, and wearing a huge ear-to-ear grin. Still too weak to walk or even feed herself, she nevertheless knew she had passed a milestone. All I could manage to say was, "Wow," which seemed to translate just fine. The next day Maria's three-year-old daughter was there when we went into her room. Her daughter looked at us and immediately buried herself in her mother's skirt, the typical reaction of a child to white coats, and Maria beamed with joy. She was definitely getting better.

After nearly two months in the hospital, Maria was discharged a few days ago, and slipped back into the shadowy life of a non-citizen. She is living with relatives in another city where we were fortunate enough to know doctors who will care for her. I will probably never see her again, but I won't soon forget her. Hopefully, I also won't forget what I relearned at her bedside: that communication is more than talking, and healing is more than prescribing medicine.

17

POSITIVE ATTITUDE

Vanderbilt's Oakley Ray, a member of the Departments of Psychology, Psychiatry, and Pharmacology, has written a most interesting piece in a recent issue of *American Psychologist*, in which he reviews the evidence regarding the role of a positive outlook on the outcomes of various diseases. While the interpretation of the evidence is still somewhat controversial, there is a strong case to be made that those with a positive outlook, and those with a significant spiritual life, fare better if afflicted with any of a variety of conditions, from cancer to heart disease, than do those without such traits or beliefs.

Dr. Ray reminds us of the seminal articles by Norman Cousins, former editor of the *Saturday Review*, on Cousins' own illness. Although a diagnosis was never firmly established, Cousins was clearly in a state of steadily declining health until he began to change his own attitude, something he attributed to humor. Cousins was so convincing that he was later named a professor at the UCLA School of Medicine, presumably to teach young doctors what he had learned about the value of positive thinking.

Though I remain somewhat skeptical about some of the studies, I am not unconvinced at all about one thing: people with a positive outlook enjoy a much better quality of life when faced with illness than those who see the glass as half empty. I have known friends and patients who struggle daily with unimaginable pain and stress, but because of their outlook they remain fully part of their families and circles of friends. They are individuals first and patients second. On the other hand, we all know people whose medical problems totally dominate their lives regardless of how trivial the problems may be. These folks see themselves not as people who have a disease, but instead define themselves by their disease.

The challenge for those of us in the medical profession is to try to deal with our patients from whatever perspective they happen to have. For the take-charge, positive person, cancer may be perceived as a challenge to be dealt with. However, in many cultures, and for some personality types, the very word has connotations almost too frightening to comprehend. Indeed, to some people, having cancer is somehow perceived as being unclean, almost like leprosy was thought of in the past. Thus comes the conspiracy of silence you sometimes witness when people are reluctant to use a word to name an illness or syndrome despite how obvious it is. Conversation in such cases becomes awkward and contrived, on occasion making it impossible for loved ones to express their feelings honestly.

Then there is the person, sometimes highly successful, who believes that God plays a day-to-day role in maintaining his or her health and material prosperity. All is fine as long as things are going well, but when faced with a major illness or other crisis, some of these individuals are suddenly overcome with guilt, anger, and doubt. In addition to the problems they already have with their physical illness, they now have the added burden of feeling forsaken by their God. These people need special attention and care.

So, while I agree in general with much of what Dr. Ray, Norman Cousins, and many others have said, I'm not sure how it affects the practice of medicine. If I had my druthers, all patients would be positive, take-charge types who, if they get bad news, deal with it while going on with their lives. Last week's *Tennessean* article about Mary Jo Dietsch, an eight-year-old Mt. Juliet girl with cancer whose positive attitude has amazed and pleased her doctors, is just such a case. Unfortunately, it seems that we can't easily teach people to develop such personality traits, and in fact these characteristics may be determined genetically or very early in life.

I do think, however, that articles like Dr. Ray's are important for doctors, nurses, and other medical professionals to read because they point out that the medical paradigm we have grown up in, one based purely on biological factors, is relatively young and certainly not universally accepted. For example, the Hmong people originally of southern China, and subjects of the 1997 book by Anne Fadiman, *The Spirit Catches You and You Fall Down,* believe that all biological events have a spiritual cause. At the other extreme may be many of those schooled in science in the past few decades, who see all illness in terms of genetics and other biological factors.

The fact is that most people fit somewhere in between, flanked by both spirituality and science. Our challenge is to find where they are and to work within that framework to bring about behavior most likely to improve their condition.

18

RESOLVE TO MAKE THE NEW YEAR
GO BY A BIT MORE SLOWLY

I don't know about you, but every year I'm grateful for the lull between Christmas and New Year's. The social activities, family gatherings, excited children, and general overindulgence of the Christmas season leave me in a state of near exhaustion, and I need a little time to get myself together before the dreadful month of January, with its short days and miserable weather. In addition, this is a good time to pause and reflect on the important events of the past year.

For me, the end of the year always brings these periods of reflection. I know the whole concept of a new year is strictly artificial, a human creation. Whether we follow the common calendar of today or the Hebrew, Chinese, or any other calendar, it seems that nearly all cultures declare a date for the beginning of the year and have some sort of celebration when each old year ends and the new one begins. So, artificial or not, the turning of the calendar is as good a time as any to take stock of things.

Increasingly, the arrival of a new year seems to come faster and faster. Maybe it's true that time flies when you're having fun, but lately it seems to be flying whether I'm having fun or not. The late Dr. F. Tremaine (Josh) Billings, who died this year, was the secretary of his Princeton class of 1933. He submitted a regular update on the class sixteen times a year. Though his later columns dealt mostly with the failing health of the surviving fifty-six members of an original class of 622, Dr. Billings wrote in 2002, "Time goes by as though telephone poles were a picket fence."

Time isn't flying by for Romy, however. Romy is my three-year-old granddaughter, and for her every day is wonderful. Although she did get a little caught up in the anticipation of Christmas, for the most part for Romy, yesterday is pretty much gone and irrelevant, and tomorrow is far in the future, though certainly eagerly anticipated. It's fair to say she totally lives in the moment. Each day is chock full of playing, learning new things, and letting her imagination carry her from one exciting fantasy to another.

And that's just as it should be. Soon enough she'll grow up and notice the passage of days speeding up, and she will look back on each fading year with a mixture of joy and sadness. There will be regrets for things she said or did, and perhaps more significantly, there will be the sudden lump in her throat when she thinks of those friends and loved ones she will never see again. It's been that kind of year for me. I look back and wish I had made one more visit, shared one more glass of wine, spent one more hour.

But the new year is not only a time for reflection; it's also a time for making resolutions. So here's my resolution for 2008: I'm going to be more like Romy. I resolve not to worry too much about what I might have done better in the past, and not to dwell too much on the future. If I hurt a relative or friend, I resolve to try to heal the wound that day. And mostly I resolve to let my family and friends know just how much I love them. After all, 2009 will be here before I know it.

19

IS THERE A DOCTOR IN THE HOUSE?

People in my vicinity have this strange habit of collapsing or otherwise becoming ill, especially when I'm traveling. Of course, they don't plan it that way, but then neither do I. As a matter of fact, in all cases so far, the people involved were total strangers, and I only met them because of the familiar call, "Is there a doctor in the house?" on board a plane, or wherever.

Now I don't want to over-dramatize this. I've never saved anyone's life in such a circumstance, as several of my friends have. I've never even been discomfited much by it, if you discount the time I stopped at a traffic accident when I was a medical student, and wound up soaking wet and covered with tiny cuts from trying to extricate a dying man from his car. With that exception, most of my attempts at helping fellow travelers have actually been pleasant. I've met some wonderful people, prevented an airplane from making an unscheduled landing, and even received a spectacular free meal for two at New York's 21 Club for my trouble.

My most recent situation occurred when an elderly woman collapsed on a long flight. Once I was fairly certain she had simply fainted, and after she came to, we struck up a conversation there in the aisle, with me kneeling, and her with her head on the floor and her feet in a seat. She turned out to be from East Tennessee and we knew a number of people in common; she even updated me on my childhood doctor in West Virginia, who later moved to Tennessee and became her physician.

But my most memorable doctor-in-the-house experience was the time I was on an overnight flight from Rio to Miami, the night I took my first sleeping pill. After ten long days visiting a Brazilian medical school, I was determined to get some sleep. I ate a light dinner, put my earphones on to listen to a nice string quartet, put on my sleep mask, and closed my eyes. Just then I heard it, a nervous voice asking, "Is there a doctor on board?"

I looked at my three hundred or so fellow passengers. No one moved, so I called the stewardess and explained about taking the pill. As I wiped my face with a cool cloth, the stewardess told me that there was a child on board with appendicitis, and the pilot was preparing to land in Venezuela.

We went to the seats of a hysterical Brazilian couple with their five- or six-year-old son, who was doubled over and crying in pain. The flight attendant explained that I was a doctor (she skipped the part about the pill), and I asked the parents to move to the aisle so I could examine the little boy. I began to feel his abdomen, using the few comforting Portuguese words I had picked up, and as I did he slowly stopped crying. As surprised as anyone, I turned to the parents, and they looked at me with total adulation. "How had I done this?" they asked with their faces. With impressive Latin emotion, the mother hugged me, and insisted that her husband and I change seats in case I was needed later. Within minutes we three were comfortably resting in our seats, the little boy's head in my lap and his feet in his mother's. None of us moved until we circled Miami. I hadn't slept a wink, and I'm still not sure what I did, but with powers like that, who could resist the call, "Is there a doctor in the house?"

20

SICK TALK

Doc, I didn't say it was a risin', I said it was a pone, but sometimes it hurts a right smart, like a risin'."

The brand new intern, fresh out of medical school in New York, Michigan or California, will look up at the patient and wonder what language he's speaking. But it's just an introduction to the South's, specifically Middle Tennessee's, colorful medical lexicon. While each region has its own colloquialisms, ours are some of the most creative, and sometimes the most un-interpretable to an outsider. The following dictionary is offered as an aid to all of our newly-arrived young doctors, to help with their orientation.

Risin'. A boil. However, most Middle Tennesseans will use the word boil when they are talking about an actual boil, preferring to use risin' to describe a degree of pain and tenderness, as in, "It was as sore as a risin'." Incidentally, Webster's actually lists one of the definitions of *rising* as a boil. So, there!

Pone. A localized area of swelling. It may be painful but is often painless, as in, "I just put my shirt on and found this pone on my neck." The word probably derives from the shape of a pone of corn bread. I'm assuming here that any reasonably civilized person knows what that looks like.

A right smart. A term with many creative uses, it describes a moderate amount of something, often pain, as in, "It hurts a right smart." For our new interns, this term would never be used to describe the most severe discomfort, say from a kidney stone or heart attack, but it isn't trivial either. Pains described this way include those from pleurisy, blood clots, and some post-operative trauma.

Smarts. Here, used as a verb, the word takes on a slightly different, more specific meaning, that of a stinging or burning pain, often involving the skin. For example, when having a local anesthetic injected, a patient might say, "Ouch! That smarts!"

Rheumatism. Aches and pains. This word on rare occasions will be used to describe serious, even crippling disease such as rheumatoid arthritis, but usually means soreness or aches and pains from old injuries, degenerative conditions, and the like. For example, one might say, "Uncle Henry's rheumatism must be acting up, 'cause he's using his walking stick today."

Hocking (or harking). Coughing, although occasionally used for vomiting. This verb specifically describes the act of coughing something up, as in, "He's been hocking up a right smart of corruption."

Clogs. Blood clots. Note to new interns: you may not always know whether the bleeding is from the lungs or stomach, but anyone who is "hocking up clogs" is seriously ill.

Born with a veil over his face. At the time of childbirth the membranes enclosing the baby usually tear away, but occasionally they remain intact and cover the infant's face. This causes no problem for the infant, but sometimes great significance is attached to it. In some cultures it is regarded as an extremely bad omen, but around here it usually is used to explain slight eccentricity, as in, "Doc, that's just the way he is. He was born with a veil over his face."

High blood. High blood pressure.

Low blood. Anemia, thus making perfect sense out of this apparent contradiction: "I've had high blood for years, but now they're treating me for both high blood and low blood."

That's just a beginning, new doctors. Welcome to Middle Tennessee. You'll love it here...once you learn our language.

II

END-OF-LIFE ISSUES

21

WIT

Wit, the Pulitzer Prize-winning play opening next week at TPAC, is the story of the terminal illness of a woman with ovarian cancer. Ten days ago the cast performed a reading of the play before an audience of medical and nursing students and faculty from Vanderbilt, Meharry, and Belmont.

It was a profoundly moving experience, and for the physicians in the audience there were many moments of discomfort. The doctors in the play are oncologists involved in clinical research, and when it comes to the care of this woman, portrayed with great skill by Tandy Cronin, they are beyond cold. They are totally clueless, to use a popular phrase. They see their patient exclusively as another addition to their research protocol, nothing more, and nothing less. It is not adequate to describe them as lacking in compassion; they are lacking in awareness, and they don't seem to know how cold and uncaring they are.

I must make one thing clear. Ms. Cronin's character, Vivian Bearing, is not what doctors would describe as a "good" patient, one who understands quickly, asks few questions, and gets on with the treatment. Instead, Vivian is a fifty-year-old, unmarried professor of seventeenth century English literature whose specialty, of all things, is the Holy Sonnets of John Donne, with their preoccupations on death.

One gets the impression that Vivian's is a life deliberately chosen, that she didn't just stumble into this tightly confined existence.

She cares passionately about words and their meanings, so as her doctors throw medical terms around willy nilly, she tries to dissect and understand every term, every gesture. As we learn, she cares not only about words, she cares about punctuation. For example, we see her remember in detail a reprimand she received as a graduate student for using a translation containing a semicolon rather than a comma in Donne's famous line, "And death shall be no more; death, thou shalt die."

What she doesn't seem to care much about is people. She has few friends (none?), and teaches one of the toughest classes in the university, where she routinely embarrasses some of her students. Her life is totally under her control, well-defined, with everything in its place. And then along come cancer and chemotherapy, research-minded doctors, and the routine and degradation of tests and examinations in the hospital. Suffice it to say that her life becomes dramatically changed. Despite her toughness, Vivian is portrayed with great sympathy as she struggles to find something to relate to as her life ebbs away. What she seizes on is irony; thus the title of the play.

After the reading I met with a small group of third-year medical students. "It's not ever like that, is it?" one asked, and from others, "I've never seen a doctor like those in the play." As we talked about the performance, the students put themselves in the role of a patient in a hospital. That patient sees her doctor maybe ten to fifteen minutes a day, unless some procedure is being performed. We spoke of how physicians communicate, of the meaning of informed consent, and of how much information people can assimilate at one time. And we talked about the role of the physician as death approaches.

Gradually the students began to appreciate something all the older physicians felt many times during the play, that we've all been doctors like those portrayed, to some degree, at one time or another. Any physician who could watch this play and not remember a patient relationship he would like to try over again is probably lying to himself. Clear communication, compassion, and understanding—these are goals rarely attained in their entirety.

I strongly recommend *Wit*. It is clever, it is funny, and it covers a topic important to us all. The Tennessee Repertory Theater cast is superb. You may not want to sit with a physician friend, however. It's disrupting to watch people squirm. As Robert Burns put it:

> Oh wad some power the giftie gie us
> To see ousels as ithers see us!

22

THE RIGHT TO DIE

When a complex medical issue is taken over by people with a narrow political agenda, the outcome is often less than desirable. Such is the situation in the recent "right to die" case involving Terri Schiavo, the Florida woman who has been in a vegetative state for thirteen years. By polarizing the debate strictly in terms of life or death, the opponents of the thoughtful court decision allowing her to die took a very complex issue and treated it as a black or white, yes or no decision. In the end, Governor Jeb Bush, with his brother's approval, overrode the courts and allowed Schiavo's feeding tube to be continued.

I sometimes envy such people. At first glance it would appear as if decision-making would be easier if we just kept everyone alive as long as we could. Easier, maybe, but wrong, both medically and morally. These cases are always tragic, but the tragedy is multiplied when we deliberately allow patients and families to continue to suffer when there is no hope for recovery.

My first exposure to this problem was in 1966, during my internship year. A mother of two, in her early forties, had collapsed in her kitchen. Her fireman husband had just been instructed in the then brand new field of cardiopulmonary resuscitation (CPR), so he called an ambulance and put his newly learned skills to work. When his wife arrived in the emergency room thirty minutes later, she was in ventricular fibrillation, a condition in which certain heart muscles tremble improperly, and which can lead quickly to death.

A single shock restored her heart rhythm to normal. We were even able to remove the ventilator the following day.

Then we settled in to the most awful six-week period imaginable. The prolonged lack of adequate oxygen had damaged her brain but, as in the case of Terri Schiavo, my patient still retained primitive reflexes that reside in the deeper parts of the brain. She could not think or carry out any volitional movements, but when her child squeezed her hand, she appeared to squeeze the small hand in response. When her husband whispered his love, her eyes sometimes turned toward him.

As the celebration of this successful CPR turned into the awful reality that was its result, we called on an older member of the faculty who was much admired not only for his knowledge, but also for his wisdom, a much less common virtue. Dr. Tumulty examined the woman carefully, and then we all met with her husband and her sister. In gentle language he explained her neurological responses as reflexes, not evidence of actual thinking, and said there was no hope of significant improvement. After further discussion we stopped the feeding tube and she died quietly a few days later, family at her side.

With better technology, our ability to keep people alive continues to improve, but the inevitable result will be more and more cases like Ms. Schiavo. We don't like to talk about quality of life as a variable in whether or not someone should be kept alive, which is understandable. On an almost daily basis I see people living with suffering that I don't know I could endure, yet they value their lives as much as I value mine, and I would never suggest that we should not do all we can to keep them functioning.

However, the part of us that is our essence, that makes humans distinct as a species, is our cerebral cortex, that thin, convoluted, very oxygen-dependent outer layer of the brain. The cerebral cortex has minimal restorative powers, and when it is severely damaged, conscious thinking, communication, and purposeful activities are lost forever. The person—the body—may still be alive, but the essence of her humanity is no more.

Two or three decades ago all states passed laws covering brain death. When there is no sign of any brain activity at all, an individual is dead. Unfortunately, total brain death is much less common than death of the cerebral cortex. It is time for rational people to address this issue, death of the cerebral cortex, with similar legislation. While zealots may be congratulating themselves that Terri Schiavo still lives, the fact is that all we're doing is prolonging suffering for all concerned.

23

THE DYING TEACH THE LIVING
ABOUT WHAT'S IMPORTANT

Belmont University president Bob Fisher and his wife Judy have carried out a most unusual study over the past few years. They performed detailed structured interviews on 104 inpatients at Alive Hospice. Many of the people interviewed were only days away from their deaths, and all of them died before the Fishers could complete the book summarizing their work. The patients ranged from children to centenarians, and their backgrounds and educational levels varied from manual workers to professors.

Their book, *Conversations with the Soon Departed—What Really Matters*, will be out in the coming months, and I recently had the opportunity to read the manuscript. I had known of their work for some time, and Dr. Fisher had very graciously accepted my invitations to speak to our internal medicine residents at Vanderbilt on more than one occasion. The lessons the Fishers learned from their interviews, while certainly important to physicians and others caring for terminally ill patients, are applicable to all of us. The Fishers are obviously deeply religious people, but the message of their book transcends even religion, at least in the usual meaning of the term. Whether religious or not, almost all the patients interviewed had concluded that love and interpersonal relationships, as the title implies, are what really matter.

In their introduction, the Fishers discuss William, a logger in his forties. Like all the others interviewed, William had found that things that were previously important to him no longer mattered at all, and instead he focused almost exclusively on his relationships with other human beings. "Don't take the small stuff for granted," he said. "And give all you can to others. Give it all and don't take nothing for granted. If a child smiles at you, smile back and know you've had a good day. If someone shakes your hand, hang on to their hand for just an instant longer than they expect."

Over and over in their interviews this same theme kept recurring. There were regrets, plenty of them, for fractured relationships, and there were amazing stories of reconciliation and peace as relationships were mended and strengthened. The patients also found great joy in small things like memories of their last family vacation. As a matter of fact, one of the interview questions asked the hospice patients what had given them their greatest joy, and the responses were almost always the same: their spouse, their children, their grandchildren.

One love story was particularly poignant. Julia, the mother of two teenagers, had amyotrophic lateral sclerosis (ALS or Lou Gehrig's disease). She had arranged to have her life support removed when her disease reached a certain point. The last thing she did as the ventilator was disconnected was to blow a kiss and wave goodbye to her beloved husband, Larry. Hours later, Larry met with Dr. Fisher and learned that Dr. Fisher was to give the commencement address at Belmont the next day. "Well, here's your speech, Bob," Larry said. "You tell those kids life is short, and you tell them to find somebody to love and hold on to them." Then he said, "Now go home and hug Judy. And when she says, 'Okay, that's enough,' and tries to push you away, don't let her go. Don't let her go."

Of all the messages to us from those near death, maybe William said it best: "Give it all and don't take nothing for granted."

24

PALLIATIVE CARE

D r. Mohana Karlekar is an outgoing, friendly woman who obviously enjoys her work. She gets to know her patients and their families, she isn't afraid to make important decisions and recommendations, and she approaches even the most difficult challenges with enthusiasm and a smile on her face. Of course, all of that could be said about lots of people, but what sets Mohana apart is her specialty, palliative care, which is the branch of medicine devoted to caring for people with terminal diseases. Mohana did her residency training at New York's Mt. Sinai Hospital, perhaps the leading institution in the country in this rapidly growing field, and subsequently she was on the faculty at both Mt. Sinai and Downstate Medical Center in Brooklyn. Since joining the Vanderbilt faculty last fall, she has established herself and her specialty as critical to our health care teams.

When I was in medical school in the 1960s, the care of people at the end of their lives received very little attention, if any. We had no instruction in either how to communicate with patients regarding fatal diseases or in the management of symptoms as death approaches. In fact, I'm sure that many more hours were spent on the addiction potential and risks of narcotics than were spent teaching us how to manage pain or shortness of breath.

All of this began to change with the rapid growth of the hospice movement. The establishment of St. Christopher's Hospice in London in the 1970s, and the publicity surrounding it, made many

Americans aware of the importance of good care at the end of life. Medicare began to fund hospice care in the early 1980s, and today virtually every community in the country is served by one or more hospice programs. We are particularly fortunate in Nashville to have Alive Hospice, regarded as among the best anywhere.

There is one problem with hospice care in the United States, however. Because of the way it is paid for, patients generally cannot enter hospice care if they are still receiving treatment, especially for cancer. So, for instance, if a patient has a disease that is usually fatal within three months, and wants to enter a clinical trial of a new drug that might prolong life a few more months, he is generally ineligible for hospice. That has resulted in increasing numbers of patients being referred for hospice care very late in their illnesses, often only days before they die, thus depriving them of the many benefits of the outstanding care hospice provides.

Palliative care is a broader concept, one that recognizes that symptom management, psychological and spiritual support, and honest communication are important whether or not the patient has exhausted every treatment option. Palliative care physicians like Dr. Karlekar approach their jobs much like any other doctor. She performs a history and physical examination, makes a diagnosis, and discusses the goals of therapy with her patient. Together they then develop a treatment plan.

A couple of months ago I arranged for Dr. Karlekar to speak to our residents. She told them about the various issues and symptoms she deals with every day. At the end of her talk I asked her to comment on her job and whether or not she found it satisfying. A huge smile broke over her face, and she said to the residents, "I love my job. I went to medical school to learn how to help people, and that is just what I do. I wouldn't trade places with anybody."

25

GAIL

I need to talk to you. Mother has a fever and is more confused."
Gail's voice was steady, but there was a sense of urgency. I have
known Gail for about four years, since the time I began caring for
her mother's rheumatoid arthritis. Gail is a confident woman with a
strong religious faith and a very supportive family. I knew that if she
said she needed help, the situation was serious.

For the past two years Gail's mother had carried the diagnosis of
Alzheimer's disease, and her deterioration had been obvious for several
months. I arranged for Gail and me to meet that morning with the
chief of pastoral care and our hospital ethicist. When she arrived it
was apparent that Gail had been crying, but she was friendly and well
composed. We began talking about her mother's values, the quality of
her life prior to the last two years, and the tragic deterioration especially
in the past six months. Gail pointed out that until then, despite a
dramatically altered personality, her mother still had flashes of her old
self. However, in recent months she increasingly had withdrawn, and
had become incontinent and largely uncommunicative.

Gail recalled incidents from the past when her mother had
encountered people similarly afflicted with Alzheimer's, and had told
Gail, "Don't ever let me linger in a condition like that." Several years
ago, after extensive discussion with her family, Gail's mother had
signed a Living Will. Therefore Gail knew precisely what her mother's
wishes were, but suddenly all of that was shaken by the reality of the
moment: her mother probably had a simple infection, pneumonia or

a kidney infection, for example, which could be treated easily by a few days in the hospital.

That is what usually happens. The pneumonia is caused by inactivity at first, but sooner or later Alzheimer's patients cannot swallow adequately, so that in addition to treating the pneumonia, a feeding tube must be used. Thus we have the situation in the United States today where an estimated fifteen thousand people in persistent vegetative states and thousands more with dementia are being kept alive by feeding tubes and even respirators.

This prospect, and the total futility of further therapy, gradually sank in as Gail talked. With little meaningful input from the rest of us, Gail concluded that prolonging her mother's suffering made no sense, neither by respirators and feeding tubes, nor even by antibiotics. After we discussed some measures to ensure her mother would be comfortable, she thanked us and left.

A few days later Gail called again. A well-intentioned nurse had implied that her mother, who was now unresponsive, might be over-sedated. Gail was angry and hurt. I decided to pay them a visit. Her mother was unresponsive and clearly dying, but the room was clean, bright, and fresh. I examined her, and as I did I thought of Tolstoy's doctor in *The Death of Ivan Ilyich*. We all knew that I was simply carrying out a ritual, but the family waited quietly as if this was something I had to do before we could have any discussion. We talked for a few minutes, Gail, her father, her daughter and son-in-law, and me. There were tears, especially from Gail's father, who had been married to her mother for sixty-six years. But there was a comforting unity in this family, based on their confidence that what they were doing was in their loved one's best interests. Despite the fact that we had plenty of treatment for the *complications* of her mother's disease, Gail knew that we had no treatment for the disease itself. Prolonging her mother's situation was not a reasonable option.

Early the next morning the phone rang. Gail's voice was peaceful, with no traces of the anger and pain of the previous day. She had just called to say thanks, and to let me know her mother had died quietly a few minutes earlier.

26

LEWIS THOMAS

Lewis Thomas died last Friday. Highly regarded within medicine as an educator and scientist, he is known to the public as the most outstanding physician-writer of our time. In books ranging from 1974's *The Lives of a Cell*, to last year's *The Fragile Species*, Thomas, more than any other writer, was able to inject humanism into cold scientific facts. His writing was so clear and well crafted that he won numerous awards for literature. Indeed, according to the *New York Times* obituary, his writing was so precise that Joyce Carol Oates often used his essays to teach her students the structure of writing.

Thomas wrote a great deal about death, both as a psychological and biological phenomenon. He noted that death, in both animals and man, is usually peaceful, as the body makes a series of adjustments that decrease pain and suffering. His own impending death from cancer was the subject of a *New York Times Magazine* interview last month. In that interview he said that dying didn't frighten him; he was confident it would be peaceful. He was troubled primarily by the inconvenience of his growing frailty, but expected his death would be as natural as anything could be, and he neither welcomed nor feared it. As surprising as it may seem to be, Thomas' attitude toward his death is actually quite commonplace. For many people the process of dying is treated as a combination of opportunity and minor nuisance.

Lewis Thomas would have enjoyed knowing Nina Thomas (no relation). When I last saw her, she was bald from chemotherapy and too short of breath to speak in complete sentences. Her legs and face were swollen, and despite her intense chemotherapy the cancer was still spreading. "This has been the best year of our lives," she said as I approached her chair. When asked what had made the year so good, she spoke of the joy of being with her children and grandchildren, the miracle of watching a garden grow, and the timeless beauty she and her husband had shared on a long-planned trip west. Although her death was certainly not welcomed, its inevitability had allowed her to concentrate on the truly important and to ignore the trivial. She died peacefully at home a few days after our conversation.

Is Lewis Thomas correct? Does the body know of its impending death and gradually adapt, so that pain and suffering are minimized? The answer, of course, is complex and intertwined with myriad religious, cultural, and psychological factors. But there are also biochemical phenomena that occur during times of great stress and pain, the most notable of which are the actions of endorphins, small molecules that are made in the brain itself and that have many complex functions, including acting almost exactly like morphine. The brain literally produces its own narcotic and thus helps decrease the awareness of pain.

Is that why aged and sick animals sometimes go off alone and die quietly? Are endorphins the reason that Lewis Thomas—and Nina and countless others—can look death squarely in the eye and grumble a little about frailty or unfinished business, but have little or no fear of death itself? The answers are elusive, and may never be fully known. In the meantime we can all take some comfort in knowing that for Lewis Thomas and many other people faced with their impending demise, death isn't such a big deal after all.

27

A HEALTH CARE PLAN
FOR LIFE AND DEATH

As I write this, my ninety-year-old aunt is being kept alive on a respirator in an intensive care unit in another city. She suffered a paralyzing stroke two weeks ago, rallied a bit, and then worsening of her chronic heart failure and other difficulties led to her present status.

Her situation is not unique. Although intensive care units were originally developed to care for acute life-threatening conditions, the fact is that elderly people with multiple chronic conditions occupy a high percentage of the nation's ICU beds.

My aunt has been ill for a long time, so long in fact, that I can't remember a time when my first question upon seeing her wasn't to inquire about her health. She had a stroke followed by carotid artery surgery over forty years ago, and gradual progression of heart failure and other problems have made her homebound for the past ten years. In addition, she's been on round-the-clock oxygen for the past several months.

We might think that in such circumstances she and her two sons would have planned for her current situation, but in my family, as in many, death just isn't discussed. We may buy a cemetery plot in advance, or pick out a funeral song or two, but frank discussions about what constitutes an acceptable quality of life, not to mention what constitutes an acceptable death, just aren't part of polite conversation.

One problem is that the movement to allow elderly, chronically ill people a peaceful death outside the ICU got caught up in discussions about resource utilization. Alarmed by the percentage of the Medicare budget spent on people in the last few months of life, health care economists looked at all of our unmet needs and concluded that we would be better served by spending those dollars elsewhere. This reached its peak a few years ago in Oregon with its health care rationing proposal, which was subsequently set aside by the federal government.

However, because of the fragmented way health care is managed in this country, if my aunt and the thousands of her generation in the same boat were taken off their ventilators and allowed to die peacefully, the dollars saved would not result in a single extra child being vaccinated, a single expectant mother receiving prenatal care, or a single case of tuberculosis receiving adequate therapy. The money simply wouldn't be spent at all.

The fact is that discussions about resource allocation are a diversion from the real issue, which is the appropriate use of life-prolonging technology. If there were any chance at all that my aunt would be restored to the well-informed, feisty, yellow-dog Democrat she always was, I would say spend the money. But that won't happen. The best she can be, and it's a very long shot at that, is a helpless, paralyzed, oxygen-dependent, incontinent, fuzzy-thinking woman who will bounce back and forth between a nursing home and the hospital until she dies in a few months.

Her lack of a properly executed Living Will presents another problem. In a strange way, the Living Will movement has created an unexpected paradox, such that the absence of such a document is often interpreted to mean there's no choice but to prolong life as much as possible, regardless of the quality of that life or the certainty of the ultimate outcome. The law of unintended consequences strikes again.

It is time to address, once again, the issue of appropriate care of the elderly, but these are discussions for society as a whole, not just the medical profession. Unfortunately, the larger society in many ways resembles my family: we know that quality of life is important, we know that what we are doing makes no sense and may be inhumane, and we just don't want to talk about it.

28

DR. PAUL MICHAEL

It is said that the curse of our species is our awareness that we will die. Whether we are alone in that or not (and some PBS programs have me doubting it), we are surely the only species to know, in many cases, the likely time and mode of our death. Doctors are both blessed and cursed in that regard. By being involved with illness and death, doctors generally appreciate the fact that we are biological creatures, subject to random diseases and injuries just like all creatures are. The curse is that sometimes doctors know too well the pain, suffering, and loneliness of many types of deaths. And doctors as patients are less likely to be comforted by comments like, "There's just a little tumor in the liver," or "Your cancer hasn't shrunk, but it hasn't grown very much either."

A friend and colleague, who happens to be my personal physician, recently learned of his incurable cancer. I have known him since he was a young resident, and I chose him as my physician because he still, in his forties, displayed the same curiosity and enthusiasm for medicine he had shown fifteen years earlier. He also has a friendly, easy conversational manner with colleagues and patients alike. I knew I could communicate with him, and figured that with our age difference, he would still be practicing as I developed the infirmities of age.

I visited him last week, not quite sure of what to expect. We had talked briefly on the phone, and he had sounded fine, but I know how involved he is with his family, how much he loved his practice, and how enthusiastic he was for his many interests including running, riding motorcycles, and accumulating one of the greatest joke collections in the Southeast.

My anxiety about our visit was totally unjustified. We began, as usual, with the latest round of jokes, and then we turned to his illness. He was totally open, discussing his physical and emotional feelings, his pride in his children, his sadness over what he will miss in their futures, the pain of having to tell his family good-bye, and the strength and support of his wife who is also his best friend. He also spoke of how focused his life is now, as he sheds all the unnecessary trappings and concentrates on just those things most important to him. This disarming honesty made communication easy and natural. Without talking "around" anything, we could both express ourselves freely.

That evening I reflected on the years I have known him and realized that I should have predicted how he would deal with a terminal illness. The people who are the angriest, the most in denial, the least able to confront their fate, are usually those with major regrets about their lives. A life lived with constant postponement of family and close personal relationships leaves an enormous gap, the perfect scenario for anger and denial. Paradoxically, that very anger and denial only widen the gulf between patient and family as death approaches.

My friend and physician is saddened, of course, by his fate, but he knows that he will be comforted by the support and love of family, friends, and patients whose lives are better because of him. He knows that legacy will last for years to come. He also leaves another legacy as he prepares for his own death, the realization that death is simply an extension of life. The best preparation for the common fate awaiting us all is a life well lived.

29

A TIME OF DYING

Publisher's note: This column was written in Dr. Sergent's regular space by Paul Michael, MD. We felt it was so significant, that it should be included.

I had my first contact with sudden death as an intern in the emergency room. The patient had literally dropped dead while sitting at supper, and there was nothing we could do to save him. Some time later, my senior resident almost jokingly asked me, "Michael, wouldn't you rather just drop dead than know you have a disease that will take you out within months?" The answer seemed obvious to me then; the opposite answer seems obvious to me now.

Six weeks ago, no longer able to play ostrich about the fatigue and lack of appetite, I broke down and actually consulted another physician. This astute clinician did not take long to get a worried look on his face after he examined me. In what seemed like just a few minutes, I was in a CT scanner, full of denial, marveling at how it felt actually to be a patient.

The news was as bad as it gets: advanced cancer of the pancreas. I recall hanging my head and listening to some sort of nebulous black noise for about a minute. When I looked up, my doctor was crying. Maybe it was the black noise, or maybe seeing the love and despair on the face of my new doctor, but a merciful event happened at that instant. I was transported back to that emergency room and was able to answer the question the resident half-jokingly posed. I had to take care of and plan for my family, and that required time. To paraphrase Thomas Kuhn, a merciful paradigm shift occurred.

I went home and told my wife the news. Her response and pain shall remain private. I became frenetic in making arrangements for my practice, my teaching responsibilities, and financial acrobatics. The paradigm shift was merciful in that it allowed me to focus on my family and their well-being without dwelling on the horror of the situation. I suspect that black noise was indeed the horror speaking to me.

There was unfinished business that proved to be the most difficult and the most painful: I had to tell my children, both on the cusp of adulthood, at eighteen and near sixteen years old.

As soon as I realized the task before me, I burst into tears and cried like an infant for what seemed an hour. It was at that moment that I realized what I feared the most about my impending death— missing the flowering of my children's lives. That evening I called my children into the bedroom and told them what had transpired that day and what it meant. I cry every time I think of that night. To see such hysterical pain in my children was more than I could bear, but as the hysteria died down, another merciful paradigm shift occurred: we all put our arms around one another and promised to make each day count, and to be open and honest about everything.

There was much growth that painful night. My son, graduating from high school soon and scheduled to go to college out of state in the fall, told us he could not leave, and would go to a local university so that he could be with his mother and sister. I realized then what a man my son had become. By evening's end, we had convinced him that it was best to stick to his original plans, and that his mother and sister were only a phone call or plane ride away. My daughter exhibited the same kind of power, offering to change schools in order to save money for the future.

The questions from the children were tentative at first, but as they realized that I was comfortable with their queries, their questions became poignant and insightful. "Dad," my son said, "I always looked forward to enjoying those things that you enjoyed with your father—graduating from college, marriage, you playing with your grandchildren." He stopped, tears streaming down his face, and mentally shifted gears. "Dad, are you afraid?"

It all fell into place when he asked that question, and I realized he had already answered it for me. "No, son, I am not afraid of dying. I am afraid of not living. I, too, will miss all those milestones you just mentioned. That is the only thing I fear." In the midst of that turmoil, I felt incredibly lucky.

Since those first few awful days, life has been pleasant and filled with wonderful moments with family, friends, and colleagues. The paradigm shift has indeed been welcome, and has allowed me to enjoy these final days with a joy for life and an appreciation for the time I have had since being informed of the diagnosis. There are still days when the despair is palpable, but those days are becoming fewer and fewer. There have even been times when I felt almost euphoric with the whole process. I find myself grasping the reality of the situation and being inebriated by the uniqueness of it. Those days are also becoming fewer and fewer.

I have been trying to write my children a series of letters, to be kept in the safe deposit box and opened on certain occasions: upon my death, graduation, marriage, and having a child. I had been unable even to start without feeling tremendous pain from the night I informed my children, and I have had to fight back the tears. Now, maybe, I can write those letters.

30

SOME END-OF-LIFE CARE PUTS FAMILIES IN AGONIZING DILEMMAS

Mary, as I'll call her, is one of those people who brighten the day. Because she lives more than two hours away and receives excellent care from her primary physician, I see her only one or twice a year. But every time her name is on the appointment schedule, I look forward to our visit.

As Mary puts it, "Mr. Right just never came along." Growing up in a small town, her vision of adulthood always included marriage and a family; but when that didn't materialize, she instead channeled her energies elsewhere, and channel she did. From her involvement in local politics, to her job as a social worker, to dozens of volunteer projects, she has made a difference in her community. But she doesn't take herself too seriously.

Every time I see her, the first few minutes are taken up by her regaling me with one story or another about the latest scandal or political intrigue in her town. So when I walked into the examination room last week, I fully expected an enjoyable update on her latest adventure. Instead, when she looked up, her face was flushed and there were big tears in her eyes.

"I've made a terrible mistake," she blurted out. Gradually she became composed and told her story. Her father had died suddenly two years ago and her mother, a strong and independent sort, had continued to live in her house alone. She was a little hobbled in her mid-nineties, but as Mary put it, she wasn't about to give up her independence. Then, three months ago her mother had a devastating stroke, leaving her partially paralyzed and unable to speak. A month later, possibly due to a second stroke, she suddenly stopped eating.

Mary and her mother had discussed this possibility many times, and Mary knew her mother wished not to have her life prolonged when recovery was highly unlikely. However, under pressure from the extended-care facility, her mother's doctors, and Mary's brother who lives in another state, Mary agreed to the placement of a PEG tube, a feeding tube that goes directly through the abdominal wall into the stomach. She visits her mother daily, and every time she sees her lying there mute, with sad eyes staring at nothing, Mary feels like her mother is crying out, "Why did you let them do this to me?"

Why, indeed? As in examples ranging from nuclear power, to hydroelectric dams, to end-of-life care, technology often outstrips wisdom. We learn how to do things, so we do them, often without adequate thought and discussion about the implications of our newest discoveries or latest actions.

Food has special significance in our culture. Virtually all religions have important prayers at mealtime and days of feasting or fasting, all of which attach deep significance to food and the act of eating, especially eating together. However, a bag containing sugar, amino acids, lipids, and assorted vitamins dripping its contents into the stomach isn't eating, it's a form of medical treatment. And like all treatments, there are some fundamental questions that must be asked: "What is the goal of this therapy? What are the risks? What are the after benefits?

Increasingly, there is a growing consensus that artificial nutrition for the demented or otherwise severely neurologically impaired simply doesn't pass the test of being a useful medical intervention. The goal, to avoid death from starvation, is replaced by death from pneumonia or some other infection, often in about the same time. The risks of such "treatment" include aspiration of the stomach contents and severe diarrhea. The benefits, if any, are pretty much limited to the possible prolongation of biological life, despite little or no chance of improved brain function.

Mary was correct that she made a mistake, but it wasn't her fault. The blame goes to those who pressured her to use this technology in the first place. Until we, medical professionals and society at large, adopt a realistic approach to care at the end of life, people like Mary are going to continue to shed needless tears.

III

SCIENCE AND MEDICINE

31

IT WAS LOVE AT FIRST SNIFF

When I was about fourteen, I was at a Fourth of July party where I began to notice one girl in particular. I had known her for a year or two, but we were only casual friends, exchanging greetings in the hallway at school and that sort of thing. That night, though, she seemed different. By the end of the evening it was as if we were the only people in the room, and when we kissed while dancing to the last record of the night, "Unchained Melody," sirens went off and cannons exploded. I was in love for the first, thankfully not the last, time.

What is it that transforms an otherwise ordinary friendship into love? We really don't know, but there are clues indicating at least some of it may be related to our sense of smell. That's right: smell. In most mammals a huge percentage of the brain is involved with the sense of smell, but compared to the very large cerebral cortex, in humans the part of the brain receiving and interpreting scents seems small by comparison. It is important nonetheless.

Closely linked to the smell centers in the brain are the areas that control our emotions, which may explain the sometimes vivid memories brought on by particular odors. For me to this day, the aroma of freshly mowed grass invariably brings back memories of high school football practice, no doubt because I spent so much time face down on the turf.

While the sense of smell in the animal kingdom has many uses, probably the most important is in mating. As far as is known, all animals produce pheromones, powerful scents that are secreted by both sexes, but especially by females at the time of maximum fertility. One only has to observe the relentless behavior of male dogs when a neighborhood female is in heat, to realize just how powerful pheromones are.

Smell is also used to select a good genetic match. Female rats, for example, can detect genetic substances in male rats' urine and will tend to breed with those whose immune systems are most compatible with their own. Similar findings have turned up in other species.

What does all of this have to do with humans? Maybe not much, since we like to think that all of our decisions, including the choice of a mate, are rational, logical products of our huge cerebral cortex. Yet it just doesn't ring true. The truth is that almost none of us can logically explain why we fell in love with the person we chose. Ultimately, it's a matter of emotion, not logic.

And that's where our sense of smell may play a role. Remember Al Pacino in *The Scent of a Woman*? He not only knew what perfume a woman was wearing, he could discern all sorts of other things, from her hair color to her emotional state. It may be Hollywood, but it also may be true.

A study by Italian researchers in this month's issue of *Human Reproduction* looked at women's sense of smell and found that it was much sharper around the time of ovulation. It doesn't take too much of a leap of faith to assume that this sharper sense of smell at ovulation helps women detect scents of male pheromones, and possibly discriminate in favor of those most genetically suitable. For women taking birth control pills, who therefore don't ovulate, there was no variation during the menstrual cycle. It might also partially explain the loss of libido experienced by some women on the pill.

The evolution of pheromones is tens of millions of years older than the development of the human cerebral cortex. Thus, it may be that we don't even recognize pheromones as scents at all, but instead simply and suddenly find ourselves emotionally and physically drawn to another person in response to a scent that doesn't register in our conscious mind.

Despite this important research and its contribution to human behavior, I would hope that there will always be room for romance. Somehow, I can't picture a teenager of the future saying, "Your eyes are like the blue of the ocean. Your lips are like rubies. And your pheromones are like fields of lilacs."

32

WHY WATCHING A SPORTING EVENT
CAN INCREASE A MAN'S SEX DRIVE

Every time the cameras panned the crowd, the behavior of the two young men a few rows in front of me became more and more outrageous. Dressed in the jerseys of their favorite team, the Titans, it was obvious they were determined to pay any price, at least within the framework of behavior just short of illegal, to see themselves on the giant screen.

The one to the right had a huge pot belly that he displayed to the wandering camera at every interruption of play, and frequently in the middle of a play as well. His slender sidekick, with nowhere near the expanse of flesh available for public consumption, preferred a series of pelvic gyrations suggestive enough to have made Elvis blush. Meanwhile, their wives or girlfriends sat together, ignored by the men except for the occasional beer break. They were deep in conversation most of the evening, seemingly oblivious to both the football game and the spectacle their men were making of themselves.

Then, as the Titans took command of the game in the second half, the unexpected happened. The men began to notice the women, and vice versa. Their cheers gradually became a foursome, and although the big one still bared his belly at every opportunity, the women became fully involved in the dancing and other gyrations.

When the game was over, both couples were hugging and cooing, obviously hoping that the evening's excitement had not yet ended.

Until last week, I would have attributed all of this to the effects of alcohol. As Shakespeare's Macduff says in *Macbeth*, "What three things does drink especially provoke?" Porter answers, "Marry, sir, nose-painting, sleep and urine. Lechery, sir, it provokes and unprovokes; it provokes the desire, but it takes away the performance."

Shakespeare knew a lot about alcohol, but last week, according to newspaper reports, researchers at Georgia State University suggested an alternative explanation for the behavior I observed. They studied fans of the 1994 World Cup soccer teams, Brazil and Italy. They found that testosterone levels of the supporters of the winners, Brazil, shot up after the win, while the poor Italians suffered a sharp decline in their testosterone.

At first glance it makes little sense. What, after all, does being a sports fan have to do with sexual prowess? Maybe, though, there's something to it. While football, unlike soccer, has never started a war, it has all the trappings of ritualistic warfare—bands, flags, even a distinction between officers (backs, wide receivers) and enlisted men (offensive linemen). To hear the fans' cries ("Kill him!" "Stomp on him!" "Hurt somebody!"), you would think you were watching actual warfare. So what does this have to do with testosterone?

Well, there may be a good evolutionary explanation for a surge of testosterone after a win. Testosterone does more than simply stimulate the sex drive. It is considered the prime reason boys are more aggressive than girls, for example. However, its main effect is on the sex drive, or libido, and that alone is enough to explain a surge after victory.

Imagine our hunter-gatherer ancestors, whose tribes were constantly bumping into one another as they searched for better hunting grounds. Given all their battles, what better way to strengthen the species than having the winners breed? And that's what they did, of course, often with the wives and daughters of the losing side.

So the next time you attend a Titans or Predators game, and some guy down front makes a fool of himself, don't get angry. Instead, relax and enjoy the spectacle, and let your mind wander back a few thousand years, and be thankful for the progress of civilization. At least he's no longer hitting his girlfriend over the head and dragging her home by her hair.

33

TELOMERES

I spent much of last week thinking about my telomeres. It was a strange week—part vacation, part attending a wedding, part visiting good friends. All the while we had one ear to the phone, waiting for a possible call from daughter Katie who is expecting our fourth grandchild any day now. Along the way, we stopped to visit our other two grandchildren and their parents, and to top it all off, in the middle of all of this I "celebrated" a birthday. Is it just me, or is time actually speeding up?

Back to telomeres, and why they were on my mind. Telomeres are a region of repetitive DNA at the tips of our chromosomes. When cells divide, the chromosomes split apart and a complementary copy, sort of a mirror image of each, is made. Thus each of the two daughter cells carries a complete copy of every chromosome, with one exception. The telomere is not completely reproduced, because with each cell division a tiny piece of the telomere is lost. It appears from scientific investigation that in a very real sense, our telomeres are our true biological clocks, ticking away until they are depleted, when our cells can no longer divide. At that point the cells begin a process called apoptosis, a form of programmed cell death.

I don't feel old, at least most of the time. I jog some, albeit much slower than in my youth. I play golf, hike, enjoy friends and family, and hope to get back to tennis when I get over recent shoulder surgery. But when I looked at the young people in the wedding party and compared them to myself and the other friends of their parents, and especially when I was around my grandchildren, I became all too aware that my telomeres are shortening and my biological clock is ticking away, whether I hear it or not.

Some strive for near immortality, hoping to extend their lives well past the century mark. A few even hope for true immortality and have themselves cryopreserved, Ted Williams style. For me, however, I think the way we're bio-engineered is about right. While I don't hope to die anytime soon, the fact is that most of us currently in our sixties can reasonably expect to be pretty active and vital until our middle or late seventies, with a few of us extending that into our eighties. Eventually, though, our shortening telomeres plus the accumulated wear and tear will catch up with us, and we'll begin to develop various chronic diseases with their resultant frailty, pain, and loss of function. That assumes, of course, that a heart attack or something else doesn't get us first.

The biggest downside to immortality is that it would take a lot out of the meaning of this life. If we remain cognizant that this is not a dress rehearsal, that there won't be another shot at life, then we should savor what is really important. Friendships, time spent helping others, time with family, and involvement in meaningful work and community activities really do matter, especially as we age. So when I try, sometimes painfully, to play on the floor with Henry and Kathryn and Emmaline, I am all too aware that their telomeres are longer than mine, and I welcome their nap times about as much as they do. But, hey, telomere or no telomere, that's some of my DNA in those little bodies, maybe even a little of my personality as well. While I don't relish becoming frail someday, I don't mind growing old. If none of us aged, I wouldn't have had the pleasure of watching my children become responsible adults and parents, and I wouldn't have had the unequaled joy of both watching my grandchildren learn and observing their personalities develop.

So, even with stiffer joints and shorter telomeres, here's to aging. As they say, it sure beats the alternative.

34

WHY SOME INFECTIOUS DISEASES ARE COMING BACK WITH A FURY

When I was a small child we would occasionally drag out old photo albums, and my parents would tell and retell stories of relatives I had never known. My paternal grandfather, for example, died when I was six months old, yet I still have a clear mental image of him based entirely on his pictures and the accompanying stories.

Some of the most vivid stories were of people who died, often quickly, from infections. An uncle I never knew died as a young man after a pimple on his face became infected. My grandmother's first husband died from a massive hemorrhage presumably due to tuberculosis.

By the time I got through medical school, I understood why they died. Infections on the face, especially those due to staphylococcus and streptococcus germs ("staph" or "strep"), can spread quickly to a major vein at the base of the brain, and cavities in the lung due to TB slowly expand, often eroding into a major artery.

In the mid-sixties, when I finished medical school, all of that seemed a distant memory. A whole new group of powerful antibiotics had been developed so that even the most serious infections, such as those involving the heart valves, could be cured in most cases. TB, likewise, was so easily treated that all the special wards and TB hospitals vanished almost overnight.

Then we saw the first warning signs that maybe things weren't as great as they first appeared. Occasional strains of staph and other bacteria always seemed to be a step ahead of even the newest antibiotics. Tuberculosis, helped by the AIDS epidemic, rebounded with a vengeance, with highly resistant strains showing up with increasing frequency.

Things only worsened in the last decade, and at the rate resistant organisms are appearing, we are rapidly approaching a bizarre sort of *Back to the Future* scenario, with people once again dying of infections that used to be easily treated. How did things get to such a state?

There are many factors—refugees, immigration, AIDS—but in the United States and other developed countries, the prime culprit is the way we introduce and use new antibiotics. We now know that resistance to a given antibiotic is almost inevitable. However, that resistance could be delayed, and in some cases prevented, if the new antibiotic were reserved for just the most appropriate cases.

What currently happens is that a pharmaceutical company develops a new drug after years of costly research. If the drug were reserved for only the most seriously ill, it might have a long and useful lifespan. However, the drug company is under pressure to make a profit as soon as possible. In addition, a competitor could introduce a better drug at any time.

So, the new drug is heavily marketed as the agent of choice for a certain problem, and while the fine print may stress that it should be reserved for the most seriously ill, that point is lost in the hoopla about its excellence in treating certain infections. A doctor treating a particular patient will often prescribe the drug, knowing that this one patient won't have much influence on the development of drug resistance. When that doctor's action is multiplied thousands of times all over the country, we are well on our way to yet another "epidemic" of a resistant organism.

The fact is that a new antibiotic should be regarded as a national and international resource, and should be handled as such. Just as there are areas of both computer science and weapons technology whose marketing and sales are tightly regulated because of national defense concerns, so should we be regulating the introduction of new antibiotics. It would require cooperation among pharmaceutical companies and between the pharmaceutical industry and the government, but similar cooperation has allowed many technology companies to remain profitable while they produce highly classified components of the defense industry.

The alternative is almost unthinkable: a world in which our grandchildren have the same fears that our grandparents did, that every cough or fever might signal the beginning of an untreatable, possibly fatal, infection.

35

HOW DO OUR GENES FIT IN
THIS BRAVE NEW WORLD?

Last week's dual articles in the journals *Science* and *Nature* about the nearly complete human genetic code have received appropriate praise and publicity for Drs. Craig Venter and Francis Collins and their respective teams. The big payoff will of necessity be delayed a few years, but it is hard to overestimate what this will mean to medicine. There will be better understanding of cancer and other diseases, improved drugs, and eventually gene therapy itself.

In the meantime, the findings are providing lots of interesting information about biology in general and evolution in particular. For example, our previous teaching had been "one gene, one protein," meaning that more complex organisms would of necessity have many more genes than less complex ones. It turns out that just isn't the case. In fact, over 95 percent of our genes have their counterpart in the mouse, leaving only a few hundred genes unique to humans. When the genetic maps of apes and other primates are decoded, they will almost surely show only a handful of genes that are not shared with humans.

In fact, one of the biggest surprises is how few genes we humans have. Previous predictions had been between fifty thousand and a hundred thousand, but the actual number turns out to be about thirty thousand. It's a tough blow for genetic chauvinists. The lowly roundworm has nineteen thousand genes and the laboratory fruit fly has fourteen thousand.

That we have so few genes is, in a way, a tribute to the amazing ability of organisms to adapt to change as they evolve. When there is need for a new process, say a metabolic pathway to adapt to change in the environment, it is highly improbable that an entirely new gene would just randomly present itself. Instead, it is more likely that the organism would "learn" new ways of coping by using existing genes and their proteins, perhaps with slight modification.

That seems to be exactly what happens. For example, the lens of the eye, the organ that caused even Darwin to stop in awe, is actually a modified form of lactic dehydrogenase, an enzyme that is fundamental to the metabolism of nearly every cell in the body. And adenosine, one of the four components of the genetic code itself, is scavenged from injured and dying cells. With the addition of phosphorous it is then converted into ATP, the primary storage form of energy for the cell.

Therefore, when we want to understand what differentiates us from a mouse, not to mention a chimpanzee, the answer is probably not a unique set of genes that determines our species, although there may be a few genes that have no counterpart. Instead, the most important differences will be the way those genes interact with one another, and it will be these interactions that likely determine the major differences among species. When one considers all the possible interactions among thirty thousand genes and their proteins, it is obvious that molecular biologists will not have to worry about job security for decades to come.

The genetic similarity among species probably should not have surprised us so much. The majority of our genes are involved in routine metabolic processes such as digestion, respiration, getting rid of toxins, etc., that are pretty much the same in all species, whether human, roundworm, or dandelion.

Consider the analogy of two factories, one that makes refrigerators and the other that builds automobiles. When you look at the individual employees (genes) you would find that most of them do very similar things in the two factories. They heat the building, unload sheet metal, operate stamping machines, paint the product, and so on. The number of people in each plant with jobs truly unique to the final product would likely be a small percentage of the total, yet the products are as different as a human and a mouse.

Determining all the ways genes interact will be center stage in the world of medicine and biology for years to come. As exciting as decoding the genome is, we will one day look back and realize that it was only the beginning of real understanding of how our genes work, not unlike the discoveries of Galileo, whose primitive telescope and creative mind combined to understand that the Earth was not the center of the universe. Reminding ourselves that it was a long way from Galileo to the Big Bang in no way detracts from the spectacular accomplishment of Drs. Venter and Collins.

36

EPIDEMIC BROUGHT ON
BY INACTIVITY, BAD DIET

I saw a patient the other day that represented my first experience with a new epidemic. It's an epidemic that will lead to thousands of Americans going blind in their thirties and forties, many more going on dialysis, and tens, if not hundreds, of thousands of premature deaths from heart disease and related disorders. If this epidemic were an infection, like AIDS, we would already be massing our resources to try to develop a treatment or vaccine, but this one is not an infection. The new epidemic is adult-type diabetes occurring in our youth.

We used to divide diabetes into two categories, juvenile and adult-onset. Juvenile diabetes, now called Type I, is caused by the absence of insulin, and is due to an immunologic attack on the pancreatic cells that make insulin. Adult-onset diabetes, now called Type II, is due to genetic factors that lead to insulin resistance. In other words, Type II diabetics still make insulin, but the tissues that insulin acts upon to allow sugar to be metabolized are resistant to its effect, thus causing blood sugar to rise.

While the genetic influence in Type II diabetes has long been recognized, it has also been apparent that other factors were involved. The most important of these, by far, is obesity. The epidemic of Type II diabetes we are now seeing in our young people is almost entirely due to the rapid worsening of the epidemic of obesity in this age group.

My first case of Type II diabetes in the young was a seventeen-year-old patient who weighed three hundred pounds. With his genetic factors, he might have developed diabetes even if he were not obese, but it would probably have occurred in his fifties or sixties as opposed to his teens.

Given the fact that most complications of diabetes involving the eyes, kidneys, heart, and blood vessels take about twenty years to develop, the implications are obvious. Since there isn't and probably won't ever be a vaccine to prevent Type II diabetes, we are forced to try the most difficult approach of all: life-style modification. It's so obvious, but it will be so difficult.

For example, when I took a dietary history on my patient and his family, it turned out that his diet consisted entirely of fast foods and prepackaged frozen foods like pizza. His obviously caring and concerned mother, who has weight problems of her own, had grown up in a household where no one cooked, and she literally didn't know how. Fresh vegetables, fruits, salads and the like were as foreign to her as yak butter. Going further, I asked about his activity level, and other than playing a musical instrument, he did little else but play computer games and watch TV. No running, no swimming, no organized sports, no biking. Nothing.

When I was in high school we had mandatory physical education, and it was tough. The boys' program was run by a Nazi-like basketball coach, and we moaned and groaned our way through running stairs, doing leg lifts, boxing and playing full-court basketball. The girls (okay, I know it was sexist) all took home economics, and were equally vocal in their complaints about learning the food groups and the rudiments of preparing food. But if some of us developed exercise and cooking habits that stuck, maybe it wasn't such a bad curriculum.

We know for a fact that changing our dietary and exercise habits will prevent diabetes. An article in the February 7 *New England Journal of Medicine* looked at people with the earliest signs of Type II diabetes, and found that even a modest life-style modification—7 percent weight reduction and 150 minutes per week of brisk walking—resulted in a substantial reduction in the incidence of diabetes.

So, the epidemic is upon us, and our choice is clear. Unless we eat a healthier diet and get off the couch, in a few years the fattest nation in the developed world is doomed to be the unhealthiest as well.

37

HENRY'S DIAPER

I could no longer pretend it hadn't happened. I had managed to avoid one for three straight weeks with our three grandchildren, all under two and a half years of age, but there was no mistaking what fifteen-month-old Henry had done. I should have suspected it. I had promised Henry's mother and grandmother that I would let them sleep in, and Henry and I had been having a great morning. It was his last day visiting with us, and I had fixed his breakfast and played with him for a while, and then we had driven to Centennial Park to feed the ducks. After returning home, Henry, who is usually a perpetual motion machine, had played quietly in the corner while I stole a chance to look at the headlines, thankful for a minute's rest. Then the unmistakable proof wafted toward me: Henry had a dirty diaper, maybe one of championship proportions.

Now I wasn't one of those fathers who always handed the babies to their mother in these circumstances. I've changed plenty of dirty diapers, including those of Henry's cousins Kathryn and Emmaline. But Henry is something else. I had watched with a combination of horror and awe as his mother, Katie, managed to change him without ruining the whole room. His feet, hands, and body were twisting and flailing in all directions as Katie calmly changed him while talking to me as though nothing was happening.

Well, thanks to a distracting toy and a couple of timely wrestling holds, I got the job done with minimal trauma to either of us or to the furniture. Then, as I carried newly freshened Henry back to the porch, I thought about what a whirlwind three weeks Carole and I had been through. We were happy but tired, not least because all three grandchildren had come down with a bad respiratory infection, one at a time.

Watching a virus infection spread through a family leaves you with a sense of wonder at the power of those sub-microscopic particles. Viruses probably evolved as a way of spreading genetic material from cell to cell, much as our mitochondria were once free-living organisms but then adapted to permanent life in our cells. In the case of viruses, it may be, as the late Lewis Thomas surmised in *The Lives of a Cell,* that the fact that they sometimes cause disease is aberrant, a byproduct of their very important role in moving genetic material around from nucleus to nucleus.

That knowledge is little comfort when actually dealing with the problem at hand: a crying child with tonsils swollen so greatly that breathing is difficult and very noisy. Knowing that the virus has no intellect and no ability to wish ill on anyone, that it was simply doing its job, just didn't help me feel any better at one a.m.

In a sense, I guess you could say that a virus infection is kind of like Henry's dirty diaper. The gastrointestinal tract is a remarkable machine for breaking down food into its constituent nutrients and then absorbing them into the bloodstream. However, just as the infectious virus may be a necessary result of a fundamentally important function, the mixing of genetic material, so is Henry's dirty diaper the necessary result of a healthy gastrointestinal tract.

All that may be true, but no matter how I rationalize it, I'll take a pass next time on catching Kathryn's cold and on changing Henry's diaper. Thanks just the same, but it's only fair to let others have first-hand experience in virology and gastrointestinal physiology. Why should I have all the fun?

38

Harvard Medical School graduate Bill Frist is in the unique position of being a potential force for science and reason on the issues of the day. Although his support of broader stem cell research was a positive step, his recent endorsement of President George W. Bush's support for the teaching of so-called "intelligent design" along with Darwinian evolution is a huge step backward. It's as if the senator checked his scientific credentials instead of his coat in the Senate cloakroom.

Charles Darwin, so revered in his home country that his likeness is on the ten-pound note, looked at the world around him and made countless careful observations, at one point even dissecting thousands of barnacle species in an effort to understand how each adapted to its environment. But it was at Galapagos that Darwin noted the unique species that had adapted to those isolated islands. As he studied them, he realized that they were related to more familiar species elsewhere and shared a common ancestor, but had evolved in different ways because of the unique environment in which they lived.

Darwin proposed that genetic mutations occurred all the time, and that occasionally certain ones gained advantages and would therefore be reproduced. He said as a species migrated and faced different environments, the adaptations gradually differentiated them so much from the original group that they could no longer breed with each other, and were thus a new species. With the explosion in understanding of genetics and molecular biology, evolution is now the fundamental principle of modern biology.

Standing against this are the proponents of so-called "intelligent design," which is nothing more than creationism with a politically correct label. Intelligent design didn't come about through rigorous scientific analysis or through an understanding of molecular biology. Intelligent design has neither testable hypothesis, nor theory that can be challenged or corroborated.

Imagine a classroom endorsed by the president and the majority leader. Say a high school teacher is discussing the explosion of mammalian species after the extinction of the dinosaurs. The teacher might first offer the evolutionary explanation as follows: The mammals living at the time of the dinosaurs were small, mostly burrowing animals, practically insignificant in a world ruled by the dinosaurs. Then a large meteorite hit the Yucatan peninsula about sixty-five million years ago, causing so much dust in the atmosphere that it blocked sunlight and produced a prolonged ice age, giving small mammals an advantage. They were warm-blooded and did not require the environment to maintain their metabolism, and they were small and did not require huge amounts of food. When the dinosaurs disappeared, the mammals were poised to fill the niches, and they did just that, evolving into the amazing variety of current and extinct mammalian species. If the teacher does as the president and majority leader propose, he presumably would then go through the whole presentation again, this time describing how the "intelligent designer" caused the meteorite in the first place. Whatever you call it, it's not science and it doesn't belong in the science classroom.

Of course, none of this would matter if it weren't for human evolution and the ultimate goal of the neo-creationists, which is to get human evolution out of the curriculum entirely. They don't care if oak trees evolved from tiny plants or if whales evolved from land-dwelling mammals. What sticks in their craw is the evidence that we, too, evolved from a common ancestor shared by the great apes and the other protohuman species, including our close relatives, the

Neanderthals, who died out only thirty thousand years ago. How would the teacher of intelligent design handle this? Were the other protohumans just experimental trials, later scrapped in place of the "better designed" *Homo sapiens*? Was the intelligent designer not so intelligent after all, or did he (or she) just employ a sense of humor to play with our minds by designing these now extinct species that can only be explained (scientifically) by evolution and natural selection?

The fact that many people believe in intelligent design is all the more reason for scientifically literate people like Bill Frist to be a force for reason. How many people believed Galileo when he pointed out that the Earth revolved around the sun? Putting so-called intelligent design into the science curriculum will accomplish nothing other than causing confusion in the minds of students and fear in the minds of their teachers.

39

FALLING IN LOVE WITH YOUR GENES

What does it take to fall in love? We don't know yet, but we may very soon. One of the unexpected spin-offs of modern genetics is that we are finding genes for things we didn't anticipate. In addition to genes responsible for thousands of normal bodily functions, and abnormal genes responsible for hundreds of diseases, genes are now being discovered that are linked to specific behaviors. For example, scientists have recently uncovered a gene for the willingness to take risks, of all things.

The progress of science, of course, is not a straight line. Instead, research observations seem to trickle in for years or decades with the apparent speed of a snail. Then, sometimes due to a technological improvement but often through a novel, out-of-the-box way of examining the facts, a new scientific theory is born. Following the development of the new theory, there is generally an explosion of fresh knowledge as the theory is tested and refined. The theories proposed by Galileo, Newton, Darwin, and Einstein are all regarded as seminal, but each was based on years of study and observation.

So it is with genetics. For example, the first person to describe DNA as the genetic material was a somewhat obscure biochemist named Oswald Avery, who later found his way to Vanderbilt and is buried in Nashville. In the early 1940s, Dr. Avery, then at the Rockefeller University in New York, stated that our genes were made of DNA, a complex sugar. However, because that ran counter to the prevailing thought, he received little fame. A decade later, Watson and Crick won the Nobel Prize for defining the structure of DNA.

For the next twenty years or so genetics made some progress, to be sure, but it was largely descriptive. Scientists recognized the major diseases associated with visibly abnormal chromosomes, such as Down syndrome, but actual gene function was poorly understood.

We now know that each gene is a segment of DNA, located on one of our forty-six chromosomes, and is responsible for production of a single protein. It was the development and refinement of the "one gene-one protein" theory that gave rise to much of modern genetics. The protein produced may be involved in forming a structure such as bone or tendon, it may be an integral part of a cell such as the cell membrane, or it may be an enzyme responsible for a biochemical reaction.

Armed with the tools of modern molecular biology, scientists from around the world involved in the Human Genome Project have set out to define the precise location and function of each of our fifty thousand* or more genes, composed of four billion pairs of DNA units. The project has been compared to the technological achievement of landing a man on the moon, but its ramifications could be many times greater.

This relatively new science is exciting but, as was the case with Galileo, Newton, Darwin, and Einstein, some of the results are raising major ethical and legal questions. Should health insurance companies have a right to know if you have a gene for diabetes, Huntington's disease, hypertension, or alcoholism? For that matter, should your automobile insurance company know if you carry the gene for risky behavior?

And just think of the personal ads of the future: "SWF with RB (risky behavior) gene on chromosome eight, seeks SWM with matching gene. Must also be compatible for MA (music appreciation) gene on chromosome nineteen. Send complete genetic map to Box 261 (photo optional)."

Subsequent completion of the sequencing of the human genome showed that our original estimates were off by a factor of two or more—we only have twenty or twenty-five thousand genes.

40

VICKS—A WHIFF IN THE AIR

The sense of smell must be the Rodney Dangerfield of the senses. In humans, at least, "it just don't get no respect!"

Not so in other animals. Dogs use it to define their territories, salmon use it to find their way back to their birthplace after several years and thousands of miles in the open sea, and most species rely on their sense of smell to determine appropriate times for mating. Smell is almost certainly the oldest of the senses in evolutionary development. Even primitive one-celled organisms have receptors on their cell membranes that tell the organism when something in the environment is attractive, such as food, or threatening, such as a toxin.

The brain centers concerned with smell are huge in other mammals, often occupying over half of the brain, and even in humans they are prominent and closely linked to centers for various emotions. Perhaps that is why we are sometimes surprised at the intensity of the sensations, even full images, released by some aromas.

We may watch a sunset and be reminded of others we have seen, we may taste an unusual food and compare it to similar foods, or we may hear a piece of music and be reminded of someone long forgotten. But particular odors sometimes have the power to recreate an entire past event, complete with all the accompanying feelings.

I had just such an experience recently. I walked into an examination room to see an elderly woman and was immediately aware of something in the air I couldn't identify at first, but it brought a flood of memories from my childhood. I saw myself being tucked in bed with an extra blanket over me. I felt the warmth of concerned parental hugs. I remembered runny noses, sore throats, spasmodic coughing, and fever. I even felt a little of the mid-afternoon guilt of staying home and playing, once I was feeling better, while my classmates were in school.

Then, suddenly, a long-neglected synapse in my brain fired and I remembered the aroma. My patient had a cold, and had applied liberal amounts of one of the most identifiable products of my childhood, Vicks VapoRub. To understand the importance of Vicks salve, as we called it, you have to understand my family and the eastern Kentucky culture. Never mind that science couldn't cure the common cold, that in the big picture, childhood colds are a rather minor nuisance, and that no physician to my knowledge has ever prescribed Vicks VapoRub. In my family, illness of any kind was treated, and treated vigorously.

We must have kept an enormous supply of the stuff, because at the first sniffle it was rubbed on my chest, stuck in my nose, given to me to be swallowed, and reapplied liberally during the night. By morning the bed was a greasy, menthol-laced cocoon. The smell invariably lingered for two or three days, so that it was rare to walk into a schoolroom in the winter and not detect at least a trace of Vicks salve in the air.

So, with my elderly patient sitting before me, I suddenly realized that I had been transported to another time and place and had not yet spoken to her during the three or four seconds of this unexpected reverie. Suppressing an overwhelming urge to give her a hug and tuck her into bed, I sat down and said, "Hello, Mrs. Jones. Is your cold any better?"

41

ST. JOAN OF ARC, THE WIFE OF NOAH, AND RADIATION

Anne was young, lovely, and desperately ill. A thirteen-year-old high school freshman, she had been completely well the evening before while attending a high school football game and post-game party with her friends. The next morning she didn't feel well and shortly thereafter had a shaking chill, followed by the passage of brown urine. By the time she reached the hospital that evening, she was profoundly anemic and in severe heart failure. She did not urinate again for more than three weeks and was dependent on kidney dialysis to try to save her life.

The year was 1970, and Anne was suffering from a poorly understood (at that time) illness known as hemolytic-uremic syndrome, or HUS. HUS is characterized by the rapid destruction of red blood cells; the resulting release of hemoglobin and other materials causes the kidneys to shut down. Even in 1970 we knew that HUS usually affected children and occasionally occurred in epidemics. Our treatment, then as now, was to try to support the patients through the period of kidney failure and hope that the kidneys recovered. Mortality was, and remains, significant.

I am reminded of Anne when reading about the backlash to the Food and Drug Administration approval of irradiation as a means of sterilizing beef. That's because we now know the major cause of HUS, especially the epidemic form. It's caused by a toxin released from a bacteria known as E.coli 0157:H7. E.coli is a natural inhabitant of the digestive tracts of humans—and cows—and very difficult to detect.

The opposition to irradiated meat seems to be due to confusion between two similar words. Just as 10 percent of Americans believe Joan of Arc was Noah's wife, according to a recent poll reported in the *New York Times Magazine,* it's not too surprising that a lot more people confuse "irradiated" with "radioactive."

Irradiated meat is meat that has been treated with low doses of X-rays, enough to kill bacteria but not enough to cook or otherwise alter the meat. X-rays are a form of electromagnetic radiation, part of a spectrum that includes visible light, radio waves, microwaves, and gamma rays. Each of these forms of energy has its own characteristics, and X-rays pass through some materials impenetrable by light, a property we use in diagnostic radiology and in radiation oncology.

Radioactive substances, on the other hand, are elements that release radiation spontaneously. These also have applications in medicine, primarily in various diagnostic scans. There are naturally radioactive substances, such as uranium, but most are man-made, using the principles of high-energy physics.

However, just as Joan of Arc had no relationship to Noah, irradiated meat has nothing to do with radioactivity. Your mouth isn't radioactive after a set of dental X-rays, and similarly meat isn't radioactive after it has been X-rayed. In addition, the meat isn't cooked or otherwise altered by these low levels of X-rays, and both taste and nutritional value are unaffected.

Anne survived HUS and recovered completely, but some children do not, and many get quite ill as we know from recent examples such as the 1993 Jack-in-the-Box epidemic. We have the power to eliminate most of these epidemics, and other food-borne diseases as well, at no risk to us. It's time we used it.

42

LOOK AT IT FROM THE
LOWLY CICADA'S POINT OF VIEW

Hmmmmmmmmh, HMMMMMMMMH," and so it goes, as the cicadas drone on and on in their adolescent sex frenzy. What a pain!

Once every thirteen years we are subjected to about six weeks of these male cicada love calls, and by then some of us will be ready to pave the back yard. By the end of their courtship ritual, cicadas will have joined cockroaches, snakes, and spiders on the list of pests we could do without.

Of course, this is an entirely human-centric view of things, but think of it for a minute from the cicada's point of view. Like many insects, cicadas have both a larval phase and a sexually mature phase. Many insects function on an annual cycle, with most of the year spent in the larval stage, followed by a brief adulthood. Examples include butterflies, moths, and our annual "dog days" cicadas.

The problem from the insects' point of view is that many of them are regarded as delicacies, especially by birds. As they evolved, each species developed a biological strategy that would guarantee survival of its young adults. For the cicada, the period between their emergence from the ground and their maturation into egg-laying, tree-pruning adults represents a great threat to their survival.

There are a number of successful insect survival strategies. Many caterpillars, for example, use camouflage, which enables them to become the identical shade of green as the leaves on which they feed. Others, with spines and various secretions, probably don't look or taste all that delicious, and thereby deflect the interest of predatory species.

When it comes to evolutionary strategies though, the cicada might be the world champion. It has been demonstrated that many birds increase their reproductive rate following a year of plenty. Therefore if cicadas emerged by the millions every year it is likely that their avian predators would increase proportionally. The increase in birds, combined with other adverse factors such as abnormal weather patterns, might threaten the survival of the entire species.

This is why the thirteen-year cycle is such a thing of beauty. By emerging just once during this long cycle, there is no way birds could be plentiful enough to threaten the entire species. Therefore, from the viewpoint of the cicada, the thirteen-year cycle is a triumph of evolutionary adaptation.

Actually, when you stop and think about it, maybe the cicadas aren't so different from us after all. Our young are born the most immature of any non-marsupial mammal, reminiscent of the long larval period of the cicada. Human adolescence is marked by an irresistible awareness of our sexuality. Adolescent humans, like cicadas, even like to group together with their own sex—boys in cars, girls at slumber parties—and then play their loud mating songs at high volume. Is that so different from cicadas?

And as we approach old age, we like to pretend we're still young. Some of us have plastic surgery, hair transplants, liposuction, collagen injections, silicone and saline implants, usually in an attempt to attract the opposite sex. Unsuccessful cicada males who sing their little insect bodies into numbness night after night would understand. What they would give for the cicada equivalent of a facelift!

So, as you curse their incessant symphony, and as you tire of stepping over their sexually exhausted bodies, try to think of them in a new light. Think of them as amazingly well-adapted creatures that were here long before our human ancestors took their first bipedal step, and very likely will still be here even if humans destroy themselves by nuclear war or by poisoning the environment.

Maybe there's one other advantage cicadas have over us: even in old age, they seem to get by just fine in their relationships with the opposite sex. And they do it without Viagra.

43

HOW DARWIN ARRIVED AT HIS
THEORY OF EVOLUTION

Well, Kansas has eliminated the teaching of both evolution and the big bang theory from its school curricula. Students there will not be expected to understand these theories, and they won't be tested on them.

Those of us who disagree with such decisions can breathe a temporary sigh of relief that this time it's happening somewhere other than Tennessee, although it is certain that as this is written, similar plans are being made in Tennessee and other states. Alabama has already taken the step of pointing out the obvious in its textbooks: that since no one actually observed the creation, we have no way of knowing exactly how it happened.

Charles Darwin was not unaware of the controversy his theory would produce. In fact, his theory was fully developed for more than twenty years before it was published. Even then, he published it only when another scientist had developed an identical theory on his own and obligingly withheld publication when he learned of Darwin's years of work.

I doubt if many members of the Kansas Board of Education have read any of Darwin's work, but if they did, they would probably be surprised to learn that Darwin was a painstaking collector of samples who made thousands of detailed observations. For instance, in his book, *The Voyage of The Beagle*, in which he documented his three-year trip around the world, Darwin noted many things that made him question what he had been taught. His discovery of shells and fish fossils high in the Andes pointed out the fact that the Earth was very much older than the few thousand years believed at the time.

His study of the rise of coral reefs was similarly important. Since the polyp that forms reefs cannot survive more than a few hundred feet below sea level, reefs had to have formed at times when sea levels were dramatically lower, again confirming that the Earth was very old, and that its geology had changed a great deal.

Most of Darwin's work on animal evolution had nothing to do with humans, or even mammals, for that matter. He spent years categorizing thousands of species of barnacles, noting their various adaptations to different environmental factors. Much of his work in the Galapagos Islands was devoted to various species of finches, each filling an ecological void created by the lack of competing species.

Today, creationists spend much energy debunking Darwin, accusing him of creating evolution to support his own doubts about religion. It is true that he wrote in his diary that he felt estranged from God after the death of his young daughter, but he wasn't the first—or the last—to doubt God under such circumstances. In fact, Darwin was a superb scientist and he did what all good scientists do. First, he made very careful observations. Next, he developed hypotheses. Finally, he espoused a theory to explain what he had noted.

Darwin's theory is still undergoing change. While Darwin believed that evolution was a gradual, progressive process, recent discoveries suggest that evolution may occur in bursts over relatively short periods of time (tens or hundreds of thousands of years) in the face of rapid environmental change. Likewise, the explosion of new information in molecular biology has enabled scientists to follow the evolution of specific genes and to compare genes from various species, all of which adds greatly to our understanding of evolution.

We've been down this road before, where a people's religious beliefs are tied to a specific and unshakable view of the natural world. Reactions to theories offered by Copernicus, Galileo, and many others are prime examples. The tragedy of the curriculum change in Kansas is not that students won't learn the theory of evolution. The tragedy is that they won't be exposed to the process that led to it. In these cases, the losers are not so much those who see the world differently from the fundamentalists. The losers are the children who won't have the opportunity to learn how the theories came about in the first place.

44

EVOLUTION AND MORALITY

If you think Darwinian evolution is controversial when discussed in terms of physical traits like the evolution of the opposable thumb or the cerebral cortex, it gets downright explosive over the evolution of behavioral characteristics. Yet, if you accept the basic tenets of evolution, any trait that persists and is widespread among peoples likely has survival value and must have a genetic explanation.

We were having dinner with friends not long ago when this topic came up. The context was the relationship between religion and morality. Some of the people said that without religion there would be no morality, and there would be no reason not to look out only for yourself and even to act in ways that might harm others as long as they benefited you. I took the rather lonely position that morality was an innate human characteristic, and that behavior patterns that we interpret as moral evolved because they have survival value. Needless to say, neither side carried the day, so after a while we switched to other, less controversial topics, like politics.

Subsequently, I came across the work of Dr. Frans de Waal of Emory University, who studies social behavior among primates, and whose findings support my position. In numerous books and articles Dr. de Waal maintains that all social animals have to alter their behavior in order to live in groups. The advantages of group living, which include defense against other groups, are great enough that behaviors must have evolved in order to allow the animals to live together. For example, Dr. de Waal has found that chimpanzees console one another after losing a battle, and that female chimpanzees try to intervene to prevent males from fighting, even to the point of removing rocks from their hands. He even reported an example of a chimpanzee drowning in a moat in a vain attempt to save another chimpanzee, a feat made all the more remarkable by the fact that chimpanzees cannot swim.

Since we share about 96 percent of our genes with chimpanzees and they are our closest relatives, it is highly likely that our own primate ancestors exhibited traits similar to those observed in chimpanzees. If so, then genes favoring cooperation and social interaction had survival value for our species and persisted, while genes favoring isolation and aggressive behavior did not.

Humans, however, have added another layer to morality. We have religious beliefs. You can go to the most isolated area in Papua New Guinea or the Amazon rainforest, and the tribes you meet will have a well-developed set of beliefs that are more or less shared by all the members of the tribe. In fact, every civilization in history has a religion at its core. There are obvious survival advantages in having a group of people with the same religion, specifically, the greater likelihood of defending and supporting others who share the same beliefs.

Unfortunately, the downside is that we often devalue people whose religions are different from ours. Whether in the time of the early Israelites, the early centuries of Christianity, the Crusades, or the current upheavals in Iraq and Somalia, people of different religions were and still are willing to kill in order to prevail. As Dr. de Waal points out, the evolutionary advantage of moral behavior has as its flip side the willingness to go to war against those who don't share our beliefs.

45

BLAME THE AGING PROCESS ON THOSE ERRORS IN THE GENES

As Regis Philbin might say, it's not my final answer, but so far I'm not too crazy about this aging business. A couple of sets of tennis doubles leaves me so stiff I barely crawl out of bed the next day, and what I call running today would have been a slow jog a few years ago. Aging is pretty remarkable when you stop and think about it. Any six-year-old can sort out a group of adults by age, yet we know surprisingly little about the underlying mechanism. What we do know is that all animals—at least all higher vertebrates—age in much the same way. An old dog getting up from a nap looks almost identical to an old man getting up from a couch. Because aging is progressive and universal, many have hypothesized that it is genetically controlled. In other words, our aging is programmed into us at the moment of conception.

One area that has received a great deal of attention is the telomere, a little tip on each of our chromosomes. Every time a cell divides, the chromosomes are all duplicated, except for the telomere. With progressive cell divisions the telomere is gradually shortened. When it is completely used up, the cell can no longer divide and eventually dies.

Scientists examined the chromosomes of Dolly, the sheep clone, and found her telomeres are the length of her mother's, not those of a sheep Dolly's age. In fact, unless ways are found to regenerate the telomere, it may turn out that the clones of adult animals are actually born with the remaining life expectancy of the parent; thus a clone of an old animal might live only a short time after birth.

However, telomeres are only part of the story. While they might explain a theoretical maximum life expectancy, the gradual loss of telomeres does not explain the relentlessly *progressive* nature of aging. If telomeres were the whole story, we would expect people to remain "young" for many years, then quickly age and die. The fact is that aging is continuous and all of the body is affected. My heart, lungs, joints, and kidneys are all functioning less effectively than they were when I was thirty.

A study in last week's issue of the journal *Science* may shed some additional light on the subject. The authors, from the Scripps Institute and Novartis Research, found that beginning in middle age our genes develop random errors as our cells divide. These errors are progressively passed on to future generations of cells, so that by the time we are elderly we have accumulated many such errors, presumably accounting for our weaker hearts, stiffer joints, and slower digestive tracts.

Is there anything we can do about it? In the overall sense, probably not much, other than follow the advice of our mothers: don't smoke, because smokers develop premature wrinkling of their skin and accelerated heart and lung disease, and eat your vegetables, because vegetables and fruits supply antioxidants and other materials that may minimize errors in cell division.

Then again, if aging really is hot-wired into our genes, maybe that's not all bad. There is absolutely no value to our species, or any species for that matter, for lots of individuals to hang around for decades after they have raised their children. After a certain point, we become just an increasing burden on the younger, more productive members of society.

Thinking of aging as a critical part of our genetic makeup is somehow comforting. If I will never again run a six-minute mile, it's because my error-ridden genes just won't let me. And that's okay, because it's in the best interest of our species. There. My knee is still as sore as it was, but I feel better about it.

46

AUNT VERA

It's probably too late to help my Aunt Vera, but increasingly we are realizing that medical advice that is appropriate for young people may no longer apply as they get older. For example, the U.S. Preventive Services Task Force changed their recommendations for pap smears a few years ago, saying that most women over age sixty-five who have had all normal smears no longer need to have the test done. The Preventive Services Task Force was created by Congress over twenty years ago, and has issued dozens of recommendations on subjects ranging from cancer and heart disease to the use of automobile seat belts. Each of its recommendations is based solidly on evidence, not just consensus, and their findings are followed by most primary care doctors and insurance companies. Many of their recommendations call for more screening of susceptible individuals for diseases like diabetes, high blood pressure, and elevated cholesterol levels. However, increasingly the Task Force is looking at age as a factor in making its recommendations.

Along those lines, this week the Preventive Services Task Force recommended that men over age seventy-five not undergo screening for prostate cancer. It's an interesting recommendation in part because the group has not yet concluded that men should be screened for prostate cancer at all. The problem is that prostate cancer is very common but also is extremely variable in its course, especially in older men. With the advent of the PSA blood test, many men over age fifty are tested annually, and thousands have had their prostate glands removed. While it is unlikely that we will stop screening and operating on men in their fifties and sixties, the Task Force agreed that any benefits of screening, in terms of both quality of life and its length, disappear by age seventy-five. After that age, screening is probably not only unhelpful, it is quite likely detrimental because it leads to surgery and other treatment with their associated complications.

This attention on what *not* to do, in addition to what we should do, is a welcome change, especially in dealing with the elderly. That brings me back to my Aunt Vera. She is ninety-five years old, lives in a small town in West Virginia, and has been a widow for almost fifty years. She has never had a driver's license, so every day she walks to the store or church or anywhere else she wants to go. She is truly fit as a fiddle, and the only health problem she has ever had was a broken hip three years ago, from which she made an outstanding recovery.

About thirty-five years ago Aunt Vera was told that her cholesterol was elevated. That runs in our family, and her physician appropriately put her on a low cholesterol diet and a medication. He died decades ago, but Aunt Vera still rigidly adheres to his diet, forgoing ice cream and other previously prized treats. At a recent family gathering, she lamented the fact that she could not eat the meat and settled for a salad instead. While her diet is certainly a healthy one, and her longevity may in part be attributed to it, it was somehow sad to see her still so concerned about her diet that she couldn't enjoy the pleasure of a fine meal.

As a fellow member of the high cholesterol club I am also on a medication and I usually try to eat a healthy diet, but I can tell you for sure that if I make it to ninety I'll eat what I please. And I'll bet the members of the U.S. Preventive Services Task Force will, too.

IV

HEALTH POLICY

47

CIVIL RIGHTS PIONEER
TAKES ON HEALTH CARE

Rev. James Lawson spoke at Vanderbilt Medical Center last week on the topic, "Towards the Healing of Humankind." Lawson is the African American who was expelled from Vanderbilt Divinity School in 1960 after being arrested at a sit-in demonstration. His expulsion led to the resignation or threat of resignation of most of the Divinity School faculty and, I'm proud to say, several key members of the faculty at Vanderbilt Medical School including Dr. Rollo Park, the esteemed chair of the Department of Physiology. Eventually a compromise was reached and most of the faculty stayed, but the event to this day remains a source of embarrassment to the university.

Historians including David Halberstam and Taylor Branch, as well as Georgia Congressman John Lewis, make it clear that while Martin Luther King, Jr., was the most visible leader of the civil rights movement, Lawson was the spiritual and intellectual force behind nonviolent resistance as a tool of social change. For that matter, for Lawson, a pacifist, nonviolence is a way of life.

Vanderbilt has formally apologized to Lawson, and last year he was named the university's Outstanding Alumnus. This year he has taken a sabbatical from his position as pastor emeritus of Holman United Methodist Church in Los Angeles to be a visiting professor at Vanderbilt, and he gave the Dean's Lecture at the Medical School. The room was packed, with students literally sitting in the aisles, but I have to admit to a little anxiety. Most of the students were born twenty or more years after the civil rights era, and to them it's ancient history. I knew Lawson would be interesting, but would he be relevant?

It turned out I needn't have worried. Speaking softly and without notes, he didn't dwell on the past at all, other than to say that he bore no ill will toward Vanderbilt or anyone at the institution. He even expressed gratitude to the late chancellor, Harvie Branscomb, for boldly integrating parts of the university when almost all Southern universities were still totally segregated.

His address was primarily a plea to the students and faculty regarding a significant present-day issue. He spoke of the injustice of a health care system more focused on profits than on caring for people. He was visibly emotional as he cited an elderly couple in his congregation who had to mortgage their home in order to pay medical bills. He totally dismissed those who say we don't have the money to pay for health insurance for all with this question: "How can we spend $200 million a *day* in Iraq and then say we can't afford to care for our own?"

He scanned the audience and issued this challenge: You, as doctors, nurses, and other health care workers, should be leading the battle for a just and fair system that would leave no one uninsured. He made it clear that while he admires the skill of doctors and nurses, if we truly care about our patients we owe it to them to be their advocates for a system that won't impoverish them when they become ill.

Lawson spoke for about forty-five minutes. Except for his soft voice you could have heard a pin drop, and even the students in the aisles hardly moved. While the civil rights movement may be ancient history to them, no one could fail to appreciate a life of conviction and purpose. While Dr. Lawson obviously appreciates the honors bestowed upon him by Vanderbilt, it is the university, not James Lawson, that is truly honored by his presence among us.

48

REV. LAWSON KNOWS WELL
THE MEANING OF FORGIVENESS

Much has been written about the Rev. James Lawson, who was expelled from Vanderbilt Divinity School for leading the 1960 sit-in demonstrations, and who recently returned to receive the university's Distinguished Alumnus award. However, there is a little known story about Rev. Lawson that shows just what a remarkable man he is.

Lawson first met Dr. Martin Luther King, Jr., when King came to visit Oberlin in the late 1950s. Lawson was already well versed in the application of nonviolent resistance, having studied at the Gandhi Institute in India before enrolling at Oberlin. However, King's speech so invigorated Lawson that the two of them stayed up all night discussing the ferment that was taking place in the South. Lawson had planned on going to divinity school elsewhere, but King persuaded him to go to Nashville, where students were already beginning to make their voices heard.

Inspired by King, Lawson changed his plans and enrolled at Vanderbilt Divinity School, where he joined the handful of blacks on a campus still almost totally segregated. Lawson quickly organized students from Fisk, Tennessee State, and the American Baptist Theological Seminary, and trained them in the methods of nonviolent resistance. These methods included acting passively while being beaten, having cigarettes put out on their skin, and being spat upon. As Congressman John Lewis points out in his book, *Walking With the Wind*, Lawson taught them that nonviolence was not merely a tool to achieve a political goal, but instead was the way to live their lives. As Dr. King had said, "You have to *love* your enemies. Love the *hell* out of them."

As is well known, Lawson was eventually arrested for "trespassing" during a sit-in and was expelled from Vanderbilt, causing a huge uproar in the divinity school and elsewhere in the university. Lawson finished his studies at Boston University, and then returned to Tennessee, eventually moving to Memphis as pastor of a large church. He became involved in the sanitation workers' strike, and it was at Lawson's invitation that his close friend Dr. King came to Memphis where he was assassinated.

A few months after King was killed, Lawson was having breakfast with his wife and saw a picture in the newspaper of James Earl Ray in his Memphis jail cell. Lawson told his wife that he was going to try to visit Ray. Curious to see what kind of person could do such a horrible thing, Lawson wrote down some questions, then went to the jail. Ray was told only that a minister was visiting and he granted permission for Lawson to see him. Lawson recounted that when he walked into that cell, he saw the most lost and forlorn man he had ever met. He balled up the paper with his questions and put it in his pocket, and instead talked to Ray as a minister. After a while he asked if Ray would like him to pray, and when Ray's answer was yes, Lawson knelt on the jail floor and prayed. As he stood to leave, Lawson asked if Ray would like him to visit again, and Ray replied that he would.

So, over the next several months Lawson became Ray's prison minister. Following his conviction, Ray was transferred to Brushy Mountain State Penitentiary. Lawson, whose wife was from Newport, Tennessee, continued to visit Ray at Brushy Mountain from time to time when they were in East Tennessee. Several years later, Ray married a newspaper photographer who had done a story about him, and he insisted on waiting until Lawson, who was by then pastor of a church in Los Angeles, could be there to perform the ceremony.

I had lunch with Rev. Lawson about fifteen years ago, and one person in the group knew about his relationship with James Earl

Ray and asked about it. Reluctantly, Lawson told the story. He never believed in Ray's innocence, nor did he even like him very much. However, as a Christian, he loved him. In fact, he loved the *hell* out of him.

We hear all kinds of politicians and televangelists spout this and that about what it means to be a Christian. My guess is that few of them really know what a true Christian looks like. They should meet James Lawson.

49

HEALTH CARE ACCESS SHOULD BE
A BASIC RIGHT OF CITIZENSHIP

Jenny," as I'll call her, came in for a follow-up appointment the other day. You probably don't know Jenny personally, but you read about her all the time. That's because Jenny is a statistic, a faceless number. Let me tell you about her.

Jenny is an outgoing, always smiling forty-year-old, who has been badly crippled with rheumatoid arthritis since her early twenties. Yet despite gnarled, twisted hands, crooked feet, and such neck pain that she often can't sit up for more than a few minutes at a time, she has made it clear that her disease is not going to control her life. She simply refuses to give up, and her spirit is a source of great inspiration to her friends as well as to her doctors and nurses. So, I always look forward to seeing her. Besides, for the past couple of years she has finally begun to respond to some new medicines, and at her last visit three months ago, she was feeling better than she had in years. However, when she returned last week, it was quickly apparent that something was terribly wrong.

After a smile and a feeble "hello," she suddenly began crying, and through her tears she told me of her unrelenting pain and of the humiliation of having to rely on her friends to help her eat, bathe, and tend to her bathroom needs. After she partially regained her composure, Jenny told me that a couple of months ago, she had been unceremoniously dropped from TennCare because she was no longer Medicaid eligible. She had previously qualified for TennCare because she was medically uninsurable, but the fact that she has a few meager assets like an old car got her kicked out of the program.

Jenny is a college graduate and has held a number of responsible jobs in the past, but her only income now is her disability check. The drug regimen that had finally brought a measure of relief costs almost a thousand dollars per month, so when she was dropped from TennCare, she literally had to choose between food and medicine. She stopped her medicines, and within a couple of weeks her disease roared back.

We pride ourselves on our health care in this country, and it is true that our technology outstrips the rest of the world. However, people like Jenny would be better off if they lived in any other Western-style democracy because all the countries of Western Europe plus Canada, Australia, Japan, and many others have decided that access to decent health care is a right of citizenship.

Among the world's industrialized democracies, we alone have huge numbers of people without health insurance. That number is now around forty-five million and probably growing as states struggle with budget shortfalls. It is sometimes difficult to put things in perspective while history is being written. I remember one of my daughters studying segregation in the South when she was in junior high school. One night she looked up at me and asked, "Why did people let it happen?" I had no answer.

So it will be with this generation's handling of the health care needs of the poor. We smugly tell ourselves we can't afford to provide our citizens the dignity of health insurance, yet many countries with less wealth than the United States manage to do so. Maybe part of the problem is statistics. Numbers, even big numbers, don't tell the whole story. In fact, they may actually blur the fact that every number represents one individual, and by focusing on statistics we don't clearly portray the degree of pain and suffering these individuals are experiencing. In fact, we may even be pleased when we read that removing people like Jenny "cleans up" the TennCare rolls.

Well, now you know one person's story, but there are forty-five million others. Someday our grandchildren will wonder how we could have allowed this to happen. What will we tell them?

50

WHAT WOULD CHARLES DICKENS WRITE ABOUT TODAY?

While I recently re-read *A Christmas Carol* by Charles Dickens, my mind kept leaping from nineteenth century London to early twenty-first century America. Dickens paints his characters so vividly that they sometimes seem frozen in time and place, but the essential issues he wrote about are just as valid today as they were in Dickens' time. Bob Cratchit and his family, for example, could represent any of the forty-six million Americans with no health insurance. Just as Bob lived in fear over how he could care for Tiny Tim, these millions of American families know they are just one illness or major injury away from destitution. And just as Bob is innocent, so are most of those forty-six million who, through lack of education or just plain bad luck, have jobs that don't provide health insurance, at least not that they can afford. By the way, most of the uninsured are employed.

Then there is old Ebenezer Scrooge, a perfect metaphor for America. Just as Scrooge was wealthy, we are the richest country in history. Similarly, Scrooge had full pockets but an empty heart, and we look at the uninsured and convince ourselves that we can't afford to fix the problem, or that it's their own fault for being poor. "Bah! Humbug!" we say to them.

Dickens' story, though, is one of redemption. The ghost of Jacob Marley tells Scrooge that we are all destined to walk among our fellow men; that is, we must care about one another. If we don't do it while we are alive, we are doomed like Marley to do it for all eternity.

When Scrooge sees ghostly visions, we realize that it is not Bob Cratchit or Tiny Tim who is the tragic character in Dickens' story; it is actually the lonely, miserable, penny-pinching Scrooge himself. "America, take a look at yourself!" Dickens is telling us.

There are many reasons this Christmas to hope that we will fix our health care crisis, including some very good economic arguments. A healthier country, in the long run, is a more productive one. But just as Scrooge might have gotten a little more work out of Bob Cratchit if he paid him more and heated his miserable office, that isn't Dickens' message. His message is that Scrooge had to help Bob in order to save himself.

So it is with America. If we truly believe in the ideals we are so vigorously defending abroad, let's take a look at ourselves right here at home. Remember how good Scrooge began to feel as he changed? We could do the same. Our Ghost of Christmas Present shows us the reality of 16 percent of our population in the same boat as Bob Cratchit, and our Ghost of Christmas Yet-to-Come shows us that the tragic character is not Bob, but ourselves. As Scrooge redeemed himself in the end, so can we.

So before you sit down to your Christmas dinner and give thanks for family and friends, pause for just a moment and think of Charles Dickens. Be reminded that if he lived in our time instead of mid-nineteenth century London, he would surely be supporting universal health insurance to protect Tiny Tim, Oliver Twist, Little Dorrit, and all the rest of his wonderful characters.

51

HEALTH CARE CRISIS IS AS CRITICAL AS SEGREGATION

As one who grew up in the segregated South, I sometimes find myself trying to explain to my children and other young people how things were at that time. I realized at a pretty early age that black people were treated unfairly, that "separate but equal" was a sham, and that there was no moral justification for the status quo. Yet I, and nearly all white people, went about our daily lives giving little thought to the situation.

The fact is that contact between blacks and whites was minimal, and what little there was almost always had the black person in a subservient role. Later on, when I was in college, I had late night dorm discussions with friends from the Deep South. They insisted that they "knew" black people because they had been around them all their lives, unlike me. But when I questioned my friends further, I learned the black people they were talking about were almost always children of domestic workers or the like. Meaningful relationships were rare.

So, despite the fact that millions of people were suffering from our laws, we whites managed to live with ourselves by the usual techniques or rationalizations. We dehumanized black people by using ugly words to describe them. We joked about them, with the jokes usually ending up with the black person looking stupid. We told stories that blamed blacks themselves for their situation by implying a poor work ethic, dishonesty, or other faults. I can even remember my grandmother, a devout Christian, telling me that if God had wanted the races to mix, He would have made us all the same.

Today's young people just don't buy all that. They look at me and ask how in the world we allowed segregation to exist for so long. And in reality, I have no acceptable answer. However, I sometimes ask if they can think of an analogous situation in America today. Are there people who are suffering unjustly because of our current public policies, similar to how blacks suffered under segregation?

They usually stare blankly, smugly confident that their generation would not tolerate such injustice. And then I remind them of an ugly, uniquely American fact: alone among industrialized countries, the United States allows a huge proportion of its people to go without health insurance. Over 15 percent of the population, forty-six million people including as many as ten million children, do not have access to adequate health care. And the consequences are very real, resulting in poorer care for children with asthma, diabetes, and other conditions, much less preventive care, higher death rates, and even financial ruin.

That's when the conversation gets interesting. "That's just not the same," they say, or, "We just can't afford it," or, "How can we insure them if they won't take care of themselves?" I point out that the answers remind me of the things white people said in the fifties. By implying that the problem is just too big to solve, and even worse, by implying that the uninsured are somehow responsible for their predicament, we deflect the conversation from the real issue.

In many ways, the problem of the uninsured is even more complex than segregation. While most of the time meaningful contact between blacks and whites was rare, we knew who they were. With the uninsured, we can't even see them. When we go to the grocery, chances are huge that some of the people checking out in front of us are terrified of their next illness, or are being denied good preventive care for their high blood pressure or diabetes, or face bankruptcy because of medical bills, and we don't know who they are. They are truly invisible. An invisible nation of forty-six million people lives within our borders, and we don't even know who they are.

Like segregation, the issue of health care for the uninsured is fundamentally a moral one. We can argue this and that about the details, but one thing is certain. Just as our children don't understand how we tolerated segregation, our grandchildren will ask how we denied people access to good health care while living in the wealthiest country on Earth.

52

CONGRESS SHOULD OVERRIDE VETO
OF SCHIP EXPANSION

When my daughter Katie was fifteen years old, her grandparents gave her an old Oldsmobile. It was roughly the size of a tank and needed paint, among other things, but she loved it. In fact, she loved it so much that she practiced driving up and down our driveway just for fun. Our driveway is on a hill that levels out at the top. One day, several months before she was a legal driver, she got to the top and the car sped up. Due to her not-yet-developed reflexes she could not find the brake fast enough, and the car shot across the street, smashing into a small car owned by a young man who was visiting our neighbors. Needless to say, I had no choice but to pay for his repairs, although I don't think I ever adequately compensated him for the shock of watching Katie's old clunker fly across the street into his almost new but much smaller vehicle.

Little did I know that the same "new driver" scenario was to be repeated several times over the next year. There was the U-turn in front of our house directly in front of an oncoming car, the denting of all four doors on a single day, and the rear-ending of a Jaguar while fooling with the radio. Despite the cost of her several accidents, I didn't report them to her insurance company for obvious reasons. She was a bad insurance risk, and if the company knew about all of these incidents, they would have dropped her like a rock.

Health insurance works pretty much the same way. There was a letter to the editor the other day opposing expansion of the State Children's Health Insurance Program (SCHIP) for uninsured children, in which the writer said that people making two or three times the federal poverty limit should buy their health insurance "like everyone else." Unfortunately, this view is shared by many of our policymakers in Washington, who still operate under the myth that there is a robust market out there for individuals, including the self-employed, to buy health insurance at a reasonable cost. It is true that you can buy insurance if you are thirty years old and in perfect health, although even then the policy is likely to come with high deductibles that discourage routine preventive care. However if, for example, you've had a mastectomy or diabetes or rheumatoid arthritis, or if your child is asthmatic, there is simply no affordable comprehensive coverage available. Incidentally, I am proud that both of Tennessee's senators voted against the president and in favor of SCHIP expansion. As a nation we should be ashamed that eight million of our children are without health insurance.

It comes as a shock to some to learn that health insurance companies operate like…well, insurance companies. They can make a profit in two ways. First, they can dilute the risk, which is what happens with group policies. I am insured through Vanderbilt, and while those insured along with me include the occasional person who might need a liver or heart transplant, the costs for those procedures are acceptable because of the thousands of employees who are reasonably healthy. When dilution is not possible, which is the case with individual policies, the company evaluates the likely costs and adjusts the price of insurance accordingly. Health insurance companies are for-profit entities, not social welfare agencies.

The fact is that the insurance model simply doesn't work for much of the population precisely because the people who need the most health care are by definition the least insurable. It's time for Congress to put the disgrace of uninsured children behind us and pass the SCHIP expansion by a veto-proof majority.

53

WHOSE FAMILY? WHICH VALUES?

Does it ever irritate you when people co-opt the language? By using catch phrases for a host of ideas, true meanings can get so muddied as to be unrecognizable. Examples of these buzzwords are legion. They include terms like "property values," a 1960s euphemism that made segregation sound like it was based on good principles. Similarly, in this part of the country, the word "Christian" is often used to mean a conservative Christian who interprets the Bible literally.

The term that most sticks in my craw these days is "family values." I consider myself about as expert as anyone in this arena, having just returned from my aunt's ninetieth birthday party. Our six-month-old spectacularly wonderful granddaughter, Kathryn, got to meet her great-great-aunts and -uncles, one of whom came despite being in a wheelchair and having terminal cancer. Although we are scattered from coast to coast, as is the case with many Appalachian families, we have always loved and cared for one another.

Now, if that's all we meant by family values, the love and protection of our own families, that wouldn't be that big of a deal, would it? After all, even mafia kingpins are famous for looking after their bloodlines. The term family values, in fact, has to mean more than caring just for our own families; it has to mean that we value things that benefit all families. So the next time someone says he's for family values, talk about these issues: First, nothing is more crucial to families than their children. With half of the children in Tennessee on TennCare, nothing is as important to their health as a strong TennCare program. Ask if your family values advocate will support increased state funding for this critical program. By the way, by not funding TennCare appropriately, Tennessee leaves hundreds of millions of federal matching dollars on the table every year.

In addition to their health, the next most critical area regarding our children is their education. Rather than watch Tennessee drift to the bottom in education, ask Mr. Family Values if he will support a state income tax, especially if the bulk of the money will go to schools. We already pay teachers less than Kentucky, Alabama, Georgia and North Carolina, and even Mississippi is gaining on us fast. How is it good for families to have our brightest teachers lured away because of our paltry teachers' salaries?

Then there are the issues surrounding the elderly, who are obviously a vital component of our families, and are deserving of fair treatment from the rest of us. However, just as the baby boomers are set to become senior citizens, with more demands than ever placed on Social Security and Medicare, what do we do? We use the temporary Social Security surplus to create the sham of a prolonged federal budget surplus, and then use those Social Security dollars to give a huge tax break to the wealthy. My idea of family values is to support candidates who will protect Social Security and Medicare from this sort of political sleight of hand.

Finally there are programs to reunite divided families, such as Project Magdalene, the remarkable program started by Rev. Becca Stevens, that works with prostitutes. In many cases these women have been able to get jobs, further their education, and regain custody of their children. Now that's what I call supporting family values.

I know that the "family values" folks, including talk show hosts and their horn-honking followers, will say that they are talking about other things, like child pornography. But don't let them off that easily. After all, it's been a while since you heard anyone who didn't oppose child pornography, hasn't it? Instead, the next time someone tells you he supports "family values," ask him about funding education, supporting children's health, and protecting Social Security. If he begins to squirm and hem and haw, you've just uncovered another hypocrite.

54

WHY I AM OPPOSED TO THE DEATH PENALTY

No doubt about it. If my eight-year-old daughter had been raped and murdered, I would want the killer executed. My anger and hatred would be so great that I would not feel satisfied until I knew he was dead. At least that's how I think I would feel, given the immeasurable sense of loss I would suffer.

Of course, I know there are limits on my revenge. If a killer is white, and especially if he is from an upper socioeconomic class, the chances that he would face capital punishment are much lower. Then there's the matter of defense lawyers. Case after case has shown that a significant proportion of people sentenced to capital punishment had an incompetent legal defense. Conversely, after having watched Johnnie Cochran in the O.J. Simpson trial, I'm convinced that Cochran, or someone like him, could get Atilla the Hun off with maybe a year for manslaughter, probably reduced to time served.

All of this comes to mind as the state of Tennessee prepares to execute Robert Glen Coe for the 1979 murder of eight-year-old Cary Ann Medlin. It will be the first execution in our state since 1960. No one has seriously argued that Coe is innocent. He is claiming insanity, something psychiatrists appear to disagree about, and questions have been raised about the adequacy of his defense in his first trial.

But that's not really the point. Let's assume for a moment that Coe is competent, that he was fairly represented, and that he is guilty. Should he be executed? The first justification for capital punishment, that it is a deterrent for similar crimes, simply doesn't wash. Maybe in the Old West, when prisoners were convicted one day and hanged on the courthouse square the next morning, there may have been some deterrence, although I doubt it. Today, with years—sometimes many, many years—between conviction and execution, there is surely no one who seriously believes that fear of capital punishment keeps people from criminal behavior. To a young criminal, two decades in prison may as well be a lifetime.

The second justification for capital punishment, and the real reason for most of us, is revenge. But the desire for revenge can lead us to make some terrible mistakes. Just recall Anthony Porter, who at one point was two days away from execution in Illinois. His case was championed by a Northwestern University journalism professor along with some of his students. They proved Porter's innocence last January and he is now a free man. How would we feel about our sense of revenge if their proof had come after his execution?

Then there are all the other prejudices, especially race, which enter into capital punishment decisions by juries. If we look merely at the history of capital punishment in our region of the country, the fact is that for a given crime, capital punishment is much more likely if the perpetrator is black and the victim is white.

Finally, there is the religious issue. Nashville has been called "the buckle on the Bible belt" because of the large number of churches and the high percentage of people who attend church, which is among the highest in the nation. In fact, many people in our area wear bracelets and T-shirts with the letters "WWJD," to remind them to ask, when faced with an issue, "What would Jesus do?" And yet a high percentage of people in our region continue to support capital punishment, despite one of history's greatest examples of the execution of an innocent man: Jesus.

Capital punishment is unfairly applied. It is also expensive, much more so than lifetime incarceration. And it is a barbarous act, whether by electrocution, hanging, lethal injection, or any other means. For those reasons and others, all Western democracies except the United States have eliminated capital punishment.

Unless there is some unexpected legal twist, the life of Robert Glen Coe, and soon that of Phillip Workman, will be in the hands of the governor. Don Sundquist has previously proven himself willing to take unpopular stands. Here's hoping he'll do so again.

55

ADOLESCENT THUNDERBOLT OF
SEXUALITY ISN'T A CHOICE

Remember going through puberty? I don't know about you, but for me puberty was more an event than a process. Changes had been occurring in my body for a while, but my life had not really been affected very much. About all I cared about was fishing and playing baseball, until puberty hit me like a sledgehammer.

There was this backyard party a few houses down the street, and after hamburgers and hot dogs, one of the girls suggested that the kids go next door to her house to listen to music. We put on the 45-rpm records, probably Fats Domino and Nat King Cole, and after sitting around awkwardly, we decided to play spin the bottle.

Now I wasn't totally naïve. We had been playing various kissing games for a few months and I enjoyed it. I had even kissed a couple of girls spontaneously after a movie or something, but the pleasure was derived mostly from the fact that we were doing something new, something our parents probably would not have approved. No bells had rung. No fireworks had exploded. Not until that night.

After a few minutes, a girl I had hardly noticed before took the bottle and instead of spinning it, just rotated it around and pointed it right at me. Then, instead of leaning across and kissing me as we had been doing, she got up, came around behind the girl sitting next to me, sat down, and put her arms around me. I can hardly remember what happened next. All I know is that alarms went off, bells rang, and the two of us spent the next hour dancing and kissing, mostly to Harry Belafonte's "Unchained Melody," a song which to this day brings back wonderful memories. I didn't sleep a wink that night and pretty much gave up fishing forever. Even baseball became much less important.

That's what happened, but what did not happen is just as important. I did not go home and ask myself if I wanted to play out my fantasies with girls versus boys. The desire to be with girls was not something I chose; it was something that was innate, so much so that it dominated my waking hours.

I have subsequently had the opportunity to discuss these matters with homosexuals, and nearly all of them knew something was different about themselves when they went through puberty. While many of them acted as if they were attracted to the opposite sex, sometimes to the point of marrying and having children, they knew even in their teenage years that what was happening to them was not the same as what was happening to most of their friends. I have never heard anybody say that he or she just thought it over and decided to be gay.

All of this came to mind when I read a report last week about mating behavior in fruit flies. As reported in the journal *Cell* by a group from Vienna, successful mating in fruit flies is very complex, involving a series of olfactory and neurological stimuli, and resulting in a complicated song and dance before mating. However, when the scientists changed a single gene, female fruit flies adopted the entire sequence of mating behaviors typical of males, even down to the "song" they produced just before attempting to copulate with other females.

While fruit flies aren't humans, and we like to think that everything we do is the result of conscious choice, one thing the genetic revolution is teaching us is that we have a lot more in common with other living creatures than we thought. We share over 95 percent of our genes with chimpanzees, and even with fruit flies we have many genes in common. If it is true that homosexuals are not gay by choice, then it would not be surprising to find that changes in one or a few genes might be sufficient to affect our sexual orientation.

Societal attitudes toward homosexuals are complex, and include everything from teenage name-calling to self-righteous Bible thumping to varying degrees of tolerance, and these attitudes are unlikely to change any time soon. However, if it does turn out that sexual orientation is genetic, then surely that finding might at least tone down the anti-gay rhetoric. Even that would be a welcome change.

56

THE RIGHT TO CHOOSE

I had been told to call "Susan" urgently. "I'm pregnant," she sobbed as soon as she picked up the phone. As I waited for her to regain her composure, I thought about this strong-willed, resilient young woman. Susan had been referred to our clinic three years before because of progressive muscle weakness. We quickly confirmed a diagnosis of polymyositis, an inflammatory autoimmune disease of skeletal muscle which, if untreated, leads to progressive weakness and possibly death.

Though she was accompanied by her husband and two young sons on her first visit, it was obvious that her husband wasn't very supportive, and I haven't seen him since. His attractive, vibrant wife had been an asset, but, as is often the case, the prospect of a chronically ill spouse was more than he could handle. They were divorced within months of her diagnosis. Still, Susan continued to be positive and upbeat despite the fact that the usual treatments for her disease either didn't work well or caused intolerable side effects.

Finally, about a year ago we saw some improvement in her laboratory tests and she began to feel better as well. Not long afterwards she told me she had been seeing a man whom she liked a lot and who was a great friend and surrogate father for her sons. Her radiant smile had returned. She talked of travel to see friends and even planned a trip to Disney World for her sons.

All of this went through my mind as she cried on the phone. After she calmed down, she told me that the relationship had broken up a few months before, and she had stopped taking her birth control pills. Then two months ago, her boyfriend suddenly reappeared.

At this point in our conversation I almost envied moralists who see the world only in black and white. Susan was facing a very difficult decision and was asking for my help. I reviewed her medications, one of which, methotrexate, is known to cause birth defects and is absolutely contraindicated in pregnancy. One of her other medicines is part of a clinical trial and it, too, would have to be stopped if she were to continue the pregnancy. Discontinuing the medicines would inevitably lead to a rapid return of her muscle condition, almost surely resulting in permanent disability or worse.

"I have only one goal in life," she said after a while. "And that is to raise and educate my sons. I am barely able to function as it is, and I know I won't be able to do it if this disease gets any worse." Unspoken was the obvious question: How in the world could she care for a newborn baby?

Personally I am pro-choice, but I find that the moral and ethical decisions I get involved in are almost never clear and obvious. Usually they are just like this, situations in which people have to choose between two alternatives, neither of which is particularly attractive. Whether it is a decision to withdraw a patient from a ventilator, or to start a young woman on a drug that will likely cause her to be infertile, I don't find that there is a right or wrong approach for every circumstance. I see my role as one who offers explanation, education, and most importantly, support.

The next morning I called Susan to check on her. She sounded much better. She had made her decision.

57

CREATIONISM IN DISGUISE

The opponents of Darwin are at it again. Having failed in numerous legislative and legal battles to have creationism replace evolution in the teaching of biology, they now have a new ploy, under the guise of what is called the intelligent design theory. Briefly, unlike the creationists, who usually base their teachings on a literal interpretation of the first two chapters of Genesis, the intelligent design proponents acknowledge the age of the earth and the fact that organisms evolve. They just say that life is so complex that there had to be a force (God) deciding it all.

The latest battlefield is Ohio, where the intelligent design advocates are attempting to get their concepts included in the science curriculum over the strong objections of the state board of education's curriculum advisory panel. We all have a stake in this issue, because it could have a profound effect on science education for years to come.

The fundamental issue here is the distinction between science and religion. Science is the effort to understand how things work. Whether it's the law of gravity, the behavior of gases under pressure, atomic dating of geological specimens, or an understanding of the structure and function of human DNA, the role of the scientist is to understand how our universe is structured and how it functions.

Religion, on the other hand, in its proper role doesn't ask how things work; it asks why. And just as I don't go to church to hear sermons about Boyle's law or the DNA double helix, I don't want our children to go to school to hear that all around us was specifically planned and designed by God. If that's how some want to interpret the world, fine. Just don't make it part of the science curriculum.

Of course, the only issue that bothers people is that of biological evolution, specifically the evolution of humans from a common ancestor shared by chimpanzees and apes. If you think about it, $e = mc^2$ is, if anything, more profound than biological evolution, but you don't have people lined up demanding that our children be taught that God specifically pre-determined precisely how much energy is contained within each proton in the nucleus of an atom.

No, the idea that sticks in the craw of the anti-Darwinists is that one or two million years ago there lived in Africa a creature whose descendents include *homo sapiens*, Neanderthals and other proto-humans, and apes and chimps. And yet, from the science, the evidence is overwhelming. The fossil record now contains numerous examples of primates in various stages of evolution, including very early examples of our own ancestors.

Some of the best evidence, though, is obtained through DNA analysis. By comparing DNA from various species, you can not only learn how closely related they are, you can also learn approximately when in their evolution the two species began to diverge from each other. Using this kind of analysis, it turns out that we and chimpanzees share over 95 percent of our genes, and we began to develop differently from our common ancestor about 1.7 million years ago. Now, that small difference in our genes is obviously critical, probably including genes controlling the development of our large cerebral cortex and our voice box and mouth capable of speech. However, with over 95 percent agreement between our genes and those of chimpanzees, the only reasonable scientific conclusion is that we're related. That's a lot closer, for example, than the DNA of the horse and the zebra.

Biological evolution is a fact. Virtually all respected biologists agree on this point, though they argue strongly over details such as the role of environmental catastrophes caused by asteroid impacts. It's long past time to put this issue behind us and teach science in the classroom. Then, if you are so inclined, teach your religious interpretation, the "why" question, in its proper place—your church.

58

PROTECT CHILDREN FROM THE NRA

W ow! What a lucky little boy!"

Two surgeons were describing a through-and-through gunshot wound which had somehow missed any major artery, the spinal cord, and all vital organs, although there was considerable bone and soft tissue damage. Obviously he was a lucky little boy, indeed.

Then I asked how the shooting had occurred, and the story was all too familiar: the child had found a relative's gun and was playing with it when it went off. It will be remembered as a potentially tragic accident involving a very lucky little boy.

And in a sense that's correct. Loaded firearms accessible to children are literally accidents waiting to happen. In a society that is as heavily armed as ours, and is apparently going to stay that way for the indefinite future, we could assume that the thousand or so children under fifteen killed each year by firearms are just the price we have to pay for the freedom to own guns. That would be analogous to the fact that we know that higher speed limits result in more traffic deaths, but we as a society have chosen to pay that price.

With firearms, though, the issue is straightforward. In every case a loaded weapon was left in a place where it could be discovered by a child. That's it, pure and simple. It's not just the gun that causes the problem. It's the fact that the gun was accessible to a child.

At the risk of offending the National Rifle Association, some of whose members apparently want American homes to be surrounded by bazookas and machine guns, some states are beginning to take a simple, common sense approach to firearm safety, and it is beginning to pay off.

In 1989 Florida passed a law making it a crime to store a loaded weapon in a place accessible to children. Eleven other states have since passed similar laws, with penalties ranging from misdemeanors to criminal offenses.

What did the guns-at-any-price faction do? Don't hold your breath. As is always the case with attempts to license or regulate any guns, they predictably argued that this was an unnecessary intrusion on the right to bear arms (leaving a loaded pistol in a child's play area?), and that it wouldn't reduce deaths.

Last week a group from the University of Washington reported in the *Journal of the American Medical Association* on the results of these laws. They looked at all twelve states with such laws and studied deaths in children before and after the enactment of the laws. They then compared the trends to overall deaths by firearms.

What the researchers discovered was that the unintentional killing of children declined by a modest but significant 23 percent in those states that had gun safe storage laws. The greatest effect was in children less than ten. The authors of the study extrapolated their results to the nation as a whole, and predicted that over a five-year period over 250 children's lives would have been saved if all states had safe storage laws.

Safe storage of firearms is actually simple. Most state laws specify either a locked box or a trigger lock. Just as with automobile seat belts, the purpose of this law is to promote responsible behavior, not to punish offenders. As time passes, as was the case with seat belts, it is likely that the use of these safety devices will increase, resulting in an even greater saving of lives.

The twelve states that have passed safe storage laws are from all parts of the country, including four from the Southeast: Florida, Maryland, Virginia, and North Carolina. Wouldn't it be nice if Tennessee became number thirteen?

59

CELL PHONES AREN'T JUST ANNOYING; THEY'RE LETHAL

The silence was deafening. My good friend had asked for my cell phone number, and when I told him I rarely turn it on, it was apparent that he just couldn't imagine such a thing. In the awkward silence I felt compelled to explain my obviously backward ways, so I stammered something like, "Why should I go out of my way to be interrupted several times a day just for other people's convenience?" That only dug the hole deeper. "I can't believe you," he said. "What if someone really needed to reach you?"

I'm not ready to declare all-out war on the cell phone, at least not yet. I'm sure there are people, somewhere, whose lives have been enhanced by the device; however, I don't think I've met many of them. Most of my interactions with cell phones involve the phone ringing in someone's pocket just as I'm trying to understand their symptoms, the inane conversations I'm forced to overhear in waiting rooms, or the unembarrassed public airing of personal and financial details in airport terminals. "Yes, buy ten thousand shares of ABC and tell Fred I'll call him about McMillan. I'm going to fire that guy first thing tomorrow."

If people care to use cell phones in those ways, it's their business I guess, but when they use them behind the wheel, that's a different matter. I remember my grandfather's reaction when car radios became standard equipment. As a sixteen-year-old I usually kept mine on a twenty-four-hour rock and roll station, and when he got in my car, he always became visibly distressed. I tried to humor him by asking what station he preferred, and he always said the same thing, "W-O-F-F. That's my favorite station."

His point, lost on my adolescent ears, was valid then, and still is now. Driving requires concentration, and anything that distracts a driver increases the possibility of an accident. Studies have shown that talking on the phone, even with a hands-free device, increases the risk of an accident as much as driving with a blood alcohol level of 0.10, the level at which one is legally drunk. In case you don't think it's a problem, just do as I often do and walk along any busy street at rush hour. What you'll see is amazing. My rough estimate is that about one–fourth to one–third of the drivers are talking on the phone, and at least that many more are doing something equally distracting, like looking in the mirror, eating, drinking coffee, or even reading the newspaper.

For some, the cell phone has gone way beyond a useful communication tool; it has become a downright addiction. Each day as I get in my car to drive home I watch as people follow this routine: start the car, fasten the seatbelt, back out, and then make a call. On the rare occasion that I've been able to overhear the ensuing conversation, it goes something like this: "Hi, Honey. I'm in my car now, leaving the garage." Meanwhile, the driver has absentmindedly pulled out in front of a car and nearly hit a pedestrian, totally oblivious to both.

In case you think I'm exaggerating, try going to your nearest Starbucks or other coffee emporium, and watch as people drive away. Virtually all will be drinking hot coffee (at several dollars a pop), many will also be nibbling on something or smoking, and the majority will be talking on the phone. I was nearly run over recently by just such a person with coffee in one hand and a phone in the other, dialing away, steering with maybe two fingers, totally unaware of a pedestrian (me!), inches from her right front fender.

The ultimate in cell phone insanity, increasingly common, is groups of teenagers or college students walking along, all of them talking on the phone. Here you have three or four presumed friends passing up the chance for real conversation in order to have separate conversations most likely about nothing. "Yeah, I'm walking along with Jim and Bob."

If people choose to fill their days with cell phone chatter, so be it. But talking and driving is as dangerous as drinking and driving, and Tennessee should follow the lead of other states and make it illegal.

60

IMMORTALITY

Remember what it felt like to be immortal? I sure do. I was young and carefree and I guess I knew intellectually that I would die some day, but death seemed so far in the future that it was as if it would just never happen. Like most teenagers, I was also anxious to fit in, to appear mature, to be one of the group.

So, at age seventeen I started smoking. Both of my parents smoked, as did most of the other adults in our family, so smoking was part of my mental image of what adults did. Even then, several years before the 1964 Surgeon General's Report on Smoking and Health, I knew smoking was harmful. I had watched family members hack and cough their way through breakfast, but hey, I was still immortal.

By the time of the Surgeon General's report, I was less certain of my immortality. I was then a third-year medical student, still smoking, but not feeling quite so cool. I had helped care for people dying of lung cancer and emphysema, many of whom were not all that old. And I noticed some tightness and occasional coughing when I played sports. So, with solid evidence from the Surgeon General that smoking caused lung and throat cancer, emphysema, and many other diseases, I decided to stop smoking. Now if you want proof that you're not completely in charge, take up smoking for a few years and then try to quit.

I had always assumed that I could put cigarettes down as easily as I had taken them up in the first place, but it just wasn't so. Despite the constant reinforcement from being around sick people, it took a year of many fits and starts before I finally kicked the habit for good. Even at that I was better than average. In one study, only 16 percent of young people that voluntarily signed up for smoking cessation programs were able to quit.

All of this came to mind with last week's report from current Surgeon General David Satcher, formerly of Meharry Medical College. Dr. Satcher reported a very disturbing increase in smoking among teenagers, especially teenage girls. Thirty percent of high school senior girls nationwide now smoke, and the rates in Tennessee are even higher.

So, girls, pay attention. First, if you start smoking, you probably won't ever stop. Second, you greatly increase your risk of lung cancer, formerly rare among women but now the cause of more deaths in women than any other cancer, including breast cancer. Oh, I forgot...you are still immortal and don't worry about death. However, since you're not unconcerned about your appearance, let's try this approach: smoking will age you very rapidly, and if you don't believe it, take a look at the people standing outside malls and office buildings with cigarettes in their mouths. Smoking causes the skin to wrinkle much faster, and it causes gum and mouth damage, leading to loss of teeth, not to mention really bad breath. It also is associated with infertility, heartburn, thinning of the bones, congenital abnormalities in your babies, and sudden infant death syndrome, all conditions that are important even to people who don't worry about their mortality.

I know that even if parents show this information to their teenagers, it is unlikely to have much effect. The fact is that as long as smoking is portrayed as attractive and fun, gullible teenagers are going to do it. It is high time to prevent cigarettes from being marketed to our youth. The way to do that is through regulation of cigarette advertising by the Food and Drug Administration.

When this issue came before the Supreme Court, it ruled five to four that cigarettes were outside the current FDA mandate. However many officials, including Health and Human Services

Secretary Tommy Thompson, are on record as favoring legislation to allow FDA regulation of tobacco. President Bush has not yet spoken on the subject.

Meanwhile Virginia Slims has a new slogan: "Until I find a real man, I'll take a real smoke," and another American teenager starts smoking every twenty-eight seconds. You've come a long way, baby.

V

REFLECTIONS ON A LIFE

61

SCHOOL PRAYER DIVIDES CLASSMATES

The Supreme Court has spoken once again on the issue of school prayer, this time ruling that student-led prayers at events like high school football games are in violation of the Constitution. Once again, critics are calling for a constitutional amendment in order, as they put it, "to put God back in our schools." Before we rush into amending the Constitution, we should pause and remember how things were before school prayer was outlawed. We should also remember why we have the Bill of Rights in the first place.

I went to a small public high school—there were seventy-two in my graduating class—in an overwhelmingly Protestant town. Each day's classes began with the Pledge of Allegiance followed by a student leading us all in the Lord's Prayer over the PA system. During Holy Week the entire first period was preempted so that we could all file into the auditorium for an hour of music, prayer, and a sermon by a rotating group of Protestant ministers.

Actually, not all of us went to those services. Judy, one of two Jews in our class and the only one in my homeroom, sat alone in the room as everyone else marched out, and the shy, quiet Jehovah's Witness boy in the other homeroom didn't go either. Likewise, a handful of Roman Catholics who went to the public school rather than the tiny Catholic school across town, also did not participate in the Protestant services.

So, all over our school, in just about every homeroom, the one or two or three kids who already had a tough enough time as members of a religious minority were singled out as surely as if we had put a spotlight on them: "Hey, look over there. She's different from the rest of us."

Adolescence being what it is meant that not all the Jews, Catholics, and Jehovah's Witnesses stayed in their homerooms. Torn between a teenager's overwhelming need to fit in versus loyalty to their religion, some chose to fit in and marched to the services with the rest of us.

Although I have to admit that I never gave it a thought at the time, we, the majority, were inflicting a form of religious persecution on those with different beliefs. The fact that participation in the services was voluntary didn't make it any less harmful. In fact, for those who had to make a choice, it probably made things worse. Even every sporting event was opened with a prayer, one hundred percent of them by Protestant clergy. I'm sure it never occurred to anyone to invite a rabbi or Catholic priest in order to acknowledge that our school had some students with other backgrounds.

The genius of the Bill of Rights is that it was written to cover situations precisely like this. While we are governed by the will of the majority, the framers of the Constitution knew that majority rule wasn't sufficient. They recognized that majorities, even well intentioned ones, will sometimes disregard the rights of others.

I'm not sure what effect, if any, those daily devotionals, Holy Week services, and prayers before football games had on our moral development. For my part, I must admit that I listened mostly to see if the person leading the Lord's Prayer got all the words right, and before football games my stomach churned so much I could barely pay attention to the coach, much less the prayer.

That's not the point, however. Even if those prayers had a positive impact on us, they disregarded the beliefs, or for that matter, non-beliefs, of others, a clear violation of the principle of separation of church and state.

For those who believe each day should begin with prayer, maybe the Supreme Court's decision will encourage something no one could argue with: a family praying together at the beginning of the day in the privacy of their own home or church. The beauty of the Bill of Rights is that it protects that activity too.

62

THE LONELY OLD MAN AND
THE LONELY LITTLE BOY

I was lying awake in the middle of the night. A few hours earlier I had seen the Italian film, *Life is Beautiful*, a story that manages to be uplifting despite the fact that it takes place during the Holocaust. My mind wandered to other times and places, and I tried to remember when I first became aware of the Holocaust, or of Jews, for that matter. It was 1950 and my family had moved from West Virginia back to its roots in eastern Kentucky, where my father became part owner and manager of an old thirty-room hotel. For the next year we lived in the hotel and took all of our meals in its dining room.

As an only child moving to a new town, I didn't have many friends except for a cousin, but he lived a few blocks away, and at eight years old, we were too young to roam the streets at night, even in the safe confines of that little town. Therefore, after dinner and homework, I spent most of my evenings in the hotel lobby.

Many of our guests were regulars—traveling salesmen, state employees who had to make regular forays out from Frankfort, and a judge who came when the circuit court met in town.

It was before television, at least before it had penetrated very far into eastern Kentucky, so after dinner virtually all of us would gather in the cavernous old lobby. As I remember it, they seemed a pretty lonely group, most of them spending their time either sitting in the swing on the front porch, weather permitting, or slumped in the overstuffed couches reading or talking in small groups.

But the loneliest by far was Dr. Levy, a circuit-riding optometrist. The little towns around there could barely support a doctor and a dentist, and no single one of them could support an optometrist. So, Dr. Levy rented a small office across the street and spent every Tuesday night with us, presumably doing the same in four other towns.

Dr. Levy was a short, round man whose black, horn-rimmed glasses were so thick that his eyes looked like huge floating globes. He spoke with a heavy German accent, and communication for him was undoubtedly made more difficult by the many idioms and colloquialisms peculiar to our area.

At night, he mostly sat alone, reading. He rarely smiled or spoke. My father was trying to relieve my boredom by teaching me to play chess, and we would manage to get in one or two games nearly every evening.

Gradually, Dr. Levy began taking an interest in our games, and we would look up to find him sitting a few feet away, silently watching us play. One night my father was called away from a game in progress, and Dr. Levy said, "Do you mind if I make a suggestion?" Within a couple of minutes he had outlined a strategy so that I was able to checkmate my father in about five moves. From that point on, Dr. Levy became my regular Tuesday opponent and coach. He would make a move, and then go over each of several possibilities before letting me make mine. In most cases, he would show me something I had failed to take into account, which would have led to my downfall.

One evening we had been playing for a while with my father watching, when Daddy asked, "Dr. Levy, do you have a family?" I don't know why the question surprised me so, but until then I couldn't imagine that he had any existence outside of hotel lobbies. Anyway, he turned to my father and said, "Only one daughter." He pulled out his wallet and showed us a picture of a beautiful young woman. As he gazed at the picture, huge tears welled up in his magnified eyes.

As I was being tucked in bed that night, I said, "Daddy, did you see Dr. Levy? He was crying." "That's okay," Daddy told me. "Men can cry, too."

Our weekly chess sessions continued until the next summer, when we moved out of the hotel. Looking back, my friendship with Dr. Levy seemed hopelessly improbable—a young boy who had never been out of Appalachia, and a European Jew whose history I never discovered. Then again, we had one thing in common: we both knew loneliness.

63

WHEN TEACHERS DON'T
HAVE TIME TO BE THERE

When I was in the seventh grade we moved to a new town, and I found myself riding the bus every day to a small school whose students mostly were from the surrounding farms. I didn't know a soul in my grade. I soon noticed who the most popular boys were, and I tried to be their friend. When they wanted to play a game I was the first to join in, and gradually I achieved a measure of guarded acceptance.

Soon we were doing more than just playing games. The acknowledged leader of the group was a big tough boy named Larry, who made it clear to all that he was in school only because state law required it, and that he would be out of there the day he turned sixteen.

Larry loved committing small, petty offenses. At first we skipped school during study hall to go swimming in the farm pond over the hill. Later, we walked to the small store down the road, and some of us distracted the owner while Larry stole a candy bar or chocolate milk.

I had always been a good student, but by the end of the first semester I had a report card loaded with C's and maybe a B or two. And I didn't care. I was having fun.

One day in the spring I was talking in class, and Mrs. Harned, my homeroom teacher, told me to wait after class. When all the students had left, she told me I was being put in detention hall every day the next week. I was outraged. No one else was made to stay after school for talking in class. Besides, it meant I would miss my bus, thus making my mother, a teacher in the fifth grade, wait to drive me home.

Surly and defiant, I began my first solitary hour in Mrs. Harned's room the following Monday, determined to be as tough as I could. She sat at her desk grading papers, and for half an hour ignored me totally. Then she put her pencil down and in a quiet voice said, "John, these things you're doing, they're not you. You have a good mind. You read and write well, but instead of using your talent, you are sneaking off in the middle of the day, and getting in trouble."

She gave me special assignments to work on that week, and soon they were fun for me. We were studying Kentucky history, and she sent me to the library to do a report on Daniel Boone. By the end of the week I rediscovered the joy of learning, and in a few more weeks found a new set of friends.

I thought of Mrs. Harned when reading of last week's "slowdown" by Metro teachers. I know there are system-wide problems in education, and like members of the school board, I also sometimes find arguments by the teachers' union to be self-serving and counter-productive. But the fact is that the United States ranks near the bottom of industrialized countries regarding the amount of money spent per pupil in elementary and high school.

My daughter Ellen, for example, teaches in an inner-city school in another city and has thirty-six fourth-graders in a room designed for twenty. That problem can't be fixed without money. Simply saying we're out of money to pay teachers what they really deserve dodges the issue. What we are in fact saying is that teachers' salaries are not a high priority.

So, last week we saw a "slowdown" when our frustrated teachers left at the end of their last classes rather than stay for their usual after-school sessions. And somewhere in the Metro schools a potentially good student, who had fallen in with the wrong crowd, missed the chance to get the special attention that was needed just at that moment.

64

KIDS TODAY DON'T KNOW
WHAT THEY'RE MISSING

In the little eastern Kentucky town I lived in as a boy, Saturdays were special and much anticipated. For the adults, it was the day to come to town, a day of shopping for the women, and for the men, a lot of whittling and smoking on the courthouse steps.

But for my pre-teenaged friends and me, Saturdays were days of wonder and delight. We went to the movies and saw a Western serial followed by not one, but two full-length Western movies. By the time we emerged squinty-eyed in the late afternoon, we had adopted the persona of the star of the day, and practiced our quick-draw maneuver in the style of Tom Mix, Hopalong Cassidy, or our favorite, Roy Rogers.

The serials—twenty or so installments each—ended each week with the hero (always white-hatted) in some seemingly hopeless situation, such as being left unconscious in a burning building, or tied up on the railroad tracks as a train sped toward him. Then the following week, he would somehow survive, but we could feel his pain as he ran through the blazing building, or used a magnifying glass that had been cleverly hidden in his shirt pocket, to burn through all the ropes, all accompanied by the roar of the rapidly charging locomotive that grew ever larger on the big screen. We never failed to applaud loudly as he leapt free just in time.

The full-length movies were only slightly more complicated. Roy Rogers and his trusted sidekick, Gabby Hayes, endlessly got into and then out of trouble defending poor farmers from cattle rustlers, or the Lone Ranger heroically rode in from nowhere just as an entire town was being held hostage by a gang of outlaws. It just didn't get any better than that on a Saturday.

When I was about eight years old, Sunset Carson came to our town. Signs had been up for weeks, and all of us were anxiously awaiting the big event. While not as famous as Hopalong Cassidy or Roy Rogers, Sunset was still well known to us, and he was going to perform rope and pistol tricks, all live and on stage; pretty special for our little community.

About twenty-four hours before the show, I began to feel ill, and soon had a fever and a rash. By the day of the show I was sick in bed with a full-blown case of the measles. Needless to say, going to the show was out of the question. Wallowing in self-pity, I had drifted off to sleep in the late afternoon when my father came into my room and said, "Son, there's someone here to see you." I rolled over, rubbed my eyes, and there he was, bigger than life. Sunset Carson, in full cowboy regalia, was standing in the doorway, accompanied by my uncle, who had secretly arranged the visit. Sunset sat on my bed for a few minutes and talked, and as he left he gave me an autographed picture. Sick as I was, I couldn't have been happier.

The death of Roy Rogers the other day brought back a flood of memories of those simple and uncomplicated times. Roy Rogers was always perfect. Even after single-handedly breaking up a barroom brawl, his hat was in place, his kerchief was neatly tied, and his shirt had nary a wrinkle. And he didn't kill his villains; he preferred to lasso them and bring them in for their humiliation and well-deserved punishment.

If they know him at all, today's kids know of Roy Rogers only as a roast beef sandwich, and they have idols like Sylvester Stallone and Arnold Schwarzenegger, who show no remorse after annihilating entire armies of enemies with their supercharged weapons. Today's kids just don't know what they're missing.

65

AUNT EJ

I just can't throw this stuff away," Mrs. X said as she dumped out a huge bagful of bottles on the table. I looked at the collection, most of which had expired years ago and nearly all of which were medicines she was no longer taking. I explained the dangers of having old medicines just lying around the house, but she kept saying she might need them someday and didn't want to waste them. I could see that I wasn't getting anywhere, so I decided to call out the heavy artillery and tell her about Aunt EJ.

Aunt EJ, whose given name was Eliza Jane, was actually my grandfather's sister and therefore my great aunt, although I never heard her referred to as anything other than Aunt EJ, even by distant cousins. She lived across the street from my grandfather and, having no children of her own, was involved in most of our family activities. She was tight with her money. Really tight. Among other things, she continued to churn her own butter well into the 1950s. One of my earliest memories of her was seeing her in the kitchen straddling her churn with the wooden "lub-dub" sound rhythmically filling the house.

She owned and ran a little store in her small eastern Kentucky town, selling an amazing array of items ranging from small toys to clothes, all of which she had bought at fire-sale prices. There was no organization to the stuff in the store, but Aunt EJ could always go right to whatever anyone wanted. Having no organization also gave her an excuse to follow people around, being certain that not a dime was ever shoplifted from her store.

Aunt EJ was married eight times to seven different men. She buried them all, and although there were whispers about the odds of being widowed seven times, as far as we know all of the deaths were due to natural causes. Her only divorce was when one of her early husbands, maybe her first but I just don't remember, was sent to the penitentiary. I also can't remember just why he was in prison but it must have been for something serious because he didn't get out until he was an old man. The state wrote Aunt EJ and asked if she would take him in as he had nowhere else to go. Being between husbands at the time, Aunt EJ not only took him in but promptly remarried him, only to find him dead in his sleep a few weeks later. She went to her grave believing the state had sent her damaged goods.

Back to the pills. One year at Christmas one of my cousins, who was eight or nine, was staying with Aunt EJ and she woke up in the middle of the night with a stomach ache. Being a daughter of the Appalachian South, where purging is the cure for all ailments, Aunt EJ fixed her a big dose of Epsom salts. My cousin took one sip and immediately spit it out and refused to take any more. Aunt EJ pleaded with her, but it was clearly a hopeless cause.

Finally giving up on the effort, Aunt EJ said, "Well I'm not going to waste a good dose of salts." And she swallowed it in a single gulp.

I told Mrs. X this story and, with a sigh, she raked all of the bottles into the trash can and left the room.

66

A QUESTION: AND WHEN DID THEY
FALL IN LOVE?

As I write this I am sitting in what used to be my bedroom. My mother, a widow for the past eight years, died two weeks ago, and I have come back to my boyhood home in Frankfort, Kentucky, to begin the process of selling it. It's a small, three-bedroom, one-bath house, similar in size and style to most of the others in the subdivision. My old bedroom is now a small den, and we have already removed the pictures and most of the clothes. The realtor, a childhood friend, is on her way over, and before the week is over the house will be empty. I may never see the place again.

We moved here when I was eleven. For the previous three years we had lived in an apartment, and when we moved to it, the house not only didn't look small, it was huge! My bedroom, with its bunk beds, offered all the space I needed for a desk and a wall on which to hang my collection of baseball pennants—the Boston Braves, Brooklyn Dodgers, and Philadelphia Athletics, among others, along with my beloved Reds.

The house sits on a quarter-acre lot, but to my eyes it was a vast estate, large enough to throw a football, climb a tree, even pitch a tent. The subdivision was only three years old and there were no fences to speak of then, so all the yards essentially ran together. It wasn't long before I knew all the shortcuts to my friends' houses, including which backyards to avoid because the owners didn't relish pre-adolescent boys traipsing through at all hours.

My nostalgia, of course, isn't limited to the house. My mother had saved old letters, and reading them is like opening a little window into my parents' lives. There are sweet, poignant letters from my father when he was working in West Virginia and my mother was teaching school in eastern Kentucky. The year was 1937, and if America was coming out of the Depression, my parents were still in it. One letter, in fact, asks if my mother needed money, because, my father wrote her, he had four dollars left and he could give her half.

The most touching were letters to and from my Uncle Stan, the source of my middle name. I was born early in World War II, and Uncle Stan was killed on Luzon in the spring of 1945, so he only saw me once, when I was a few months old. However, he addressed his letters to me, admonishing me to be sure to tell my mother this or that, and talking constantly about the fun he would have with me when "we finish cleaning up this mess."

There is also a packet of unopened letters from my mother to him, each stamped "Deceased. Return to sender." I opened them and saw that they reflected my mother's growing optimism that the war was going to end soon, and Stan would be coming home.

Perhaps the strongest emotion comes from the sudden awareness of being the patriarch of my family, albeit a small family. All those questions I had pondered will likely remain forever unanswered: What led my grandparents to each other, when she was a widow and a school teacher, and he was ten years younger than she? What happened to all those great-aunts and -uncles? How did my parents meet? And when did they fall in love?

The death of a parent is a sobering event in many ways, and it will take me a while to sort out the mixture of emotions and memories. It will also take some time to get used to the fact that for my children, I am now the repository of their family history. Just as my parents tried, with only partial success, to describe what their lives were like during the Depression, so will I explain to my daughters the sheer ecstasy of a wide-eyed eleven-year-old running into this seemingly huge house for the first time. After all, there's no one else to portray it.

67

DAUGHTER'S WEDDING:
OOPS. WE FORGOT TO PREPARE DAD

It is two hours before my daughter Katie's wedding will begin. I am sitting ramrod straight, to avoid wrinkling my tuxedo, in the back of the church. I have nothing to do.

Upstairs is a totally different story, of course. My wife, Carole, is busy orchestrating a beehive of dressing activity and last minute rehearsing, all the while demonstrating by her confident presence that everything will be perfect. Come to think of it, that's pretty much the way it's been for several months.

When Dave called me last fall to "ask" for Katie's hand, my mind fast-forwarded to being a father-in-law. I had liked Dave from the start and as I watched Katie's love for him grow and mature, I too had grown to love him.

Dave and Katie seemed to bring out the best in each other, and Carole and I felt blessed that he was coming into our lives. As the father of two daughters, I also thought that having a son-in-law would be a pretty good deal. At last I would have someone to talk to when it's third and three on the twelve-yard line.

However, I had failed to consider just how much would be involved between Dave's phone call and the actual wedding day. For the past few months, as Katie and Carole planned detail upon detail, my significance diminished to simply being a conduit of information.

This child, who used to call me from college in the middle of the day to tell me about a lecture she had just heard, now had little more to say than, "Hey, Dad, is Mom there?" Therefore, my situation just before the wedding was not all that different from what it had been for months. It was just more dramatic.

And as if the moment is not poignant enough, now the musicians are beginning to rehearse the pieces of music Carole and Katie so carefully chose. Alone with my thoughts, I can reflect on the important events in Katie's still young life. There is no instruction manual that prepares fathers for moments like these. Many of my friends have gone through a daughter's wedding, and all spoke of the emotional impact, but it's not something that can be described adequately. Now that I think about it, though, it's not too different from so many other events in her life.

For example, how can one describe the instant bonding at the moment of birth? There I was, holding Carole's hand and trying to encourage her, when suddenly there appeared this warm, wet, crying little girl for whom I gladly would have given my life. Certainly, no one had prepared me for that. And no one had prepared me for the joy of those bedtime song sessions, as her sister Ellen and I gradually taught Katie the words of the sailing songs their grandfather had taught me. Nor was I prepared for the feeling of total inadequacy when eight-year-old Katie and I sat and bawled our eyes out over the death of Peanut, her beloved mixed-breed dog.

These and many other recollections fill my mind as the minutes tick by. I had previously been jealous of Carole, whose activity level precluded any time to be alone with her own memories. While that will come later for her, I am glad to have this time right now, even if it means that the lump in my throat sometimes feels like a rock.

In a little while Katie and I will take that short symbolic walk down the aisle, and a new phase in our relationship will begin. I know that neither of us is fully prepared for what is to come, and that there may be bad times as well as good. But as I sit alone thinking of Katie while the strains of Bach fill the church, I'm pretty sure we'll do okay—even without an instruction manual.

68

DOC, WHY DO THEY CALL IT THE "FUNNY BONE"?

Yuck!" or "Gross!" were the typical responses I received from the students after showing them a model of the spine. Needless to say, it wasn't what I expected. But then, these weren't the students I was accustomed to. My daughter, Ellen, a third-grade teacher in Nashville, had asked me months ago to come and visit her class. I agreed of course, and hardly gave it another thought until a few days before my "class." Ellen told me that one of the students had seen my picture from one of these columns, and had posted it on the bulletin board. That's when the stark reality of the situation sank in: I didn't have the foggiest notion of how to communicate with a room full of eight-and nine-year-olds.

Ellen had told me they liked demonstrations, and they liked getting things to take home, so I armed myself with a suitcase (literally) full of "things"—X-rays, surgical caps and masks, T-shirts, my model of the spine, percussion hammer, stethoscope, coloring books, and a few other items.

My lesson plan was straightforward enough. I was going to show them an X-ray, and let them identify the heart, lungs, ribs, etc., and then discuss how they work. My plan worked for about fifteen seconds.

I had completely forgotten about the energy level of a third-grader. I had barely introduced myself and put up the X-ray, before fifteen or twenty hands shot up, many waving wildly. Several times the enthusiasm to be called on to answer was so great that the student forgot the question, or never understood it in the first place.

And the answers! Sure, they each knew it was a heart or an arm bone, but the response usually involved a rambling story about some injury the student had sustained, or an injury or illness involving a friend or relative. Even then, in most cases, the answer's relationship to the question was tangential, to say the least.

Desperate to maintain some control of the situation, I tried every pedagogical trick I knew. I asked questions; I demonstrated how reflexes work; I even taught them to take their pulse (no easy task, by the way). I taught from the front of the room, from the back, and from the middle. Nothing contained the bedlam.

Gradually, I realized that control was not possible, maybe not even desirable. To these children I was a one-man field trip, and they were having fun. If I wasn't, that was my problem, not theirs. And before I knew it, I was having fun, too. I just decided to go with the flow, and flow we did, from "Why do they call it the funny bone?" to "What's your middle name?"

We checked our pulses before and after exercise—my apologies to the fourth-grade class one floor below—and most came out with pretty good numbers. There was one little girl whose reported heart rate was nearly three hundred, but she looked okay, so I let it go. When the hour was nearly up, we took a group photo. There I am, wearing several sets of "bunny ears," surrounded by twenty-five children in surgical caps and masks. About all I could think was, "They really don't pay these teachers enough!"

After I left and Ellen had easily restored order, she asked them what they had learned. One hand went up. "Miss Sergent, your daddy's a lot older than he looks in that picture."

69

IS WILL'S STORY ABOUT A MIRACLE?
YOU DECIDE

I don't believe in miracles, so overcoming adversity, medical or otherwise, cannot, in my estimation, be a miracle. However, this story about Will points out the value of mental and emotional fortitude and courage. I know that the improbable, the beating of the odds, sometimes DOES happen, and if you want to call that a miracle, it's all right with me.

Will is my cousin—more like a nephew actually, but that's another story. Will was, to put it mildly, a difficult child, and as a young adult he was well on his way to wasting his life. He had dropped out of college, and his stubbornness and temper had gotten him into trouble more than once. Dana was Will's girlfriend. A Columbian by birth, she was a warm and friendly young woman who obviously cared a great deal about Will, but try as she might, she was unable to change him, and their relationship was a turbulent and often explosive one.

Eight years ago, Dana and Will were involved in a traffic accident. Dana suffered multiple fractures and internal injuries, but she eventually made a complete recovery. Will, however, sustained a massive head injury. After weeks of being in a coma and multiple neurosurgical procedures, it was apparent that Will would survive, but with a severe handicap. One arm and leg were left virtually useless, and the other leg was weak and spastic. His speech was slow, difficult and often unintelligible.

Like many brain-injured people, Will was emotionally unstable and occasionally hostile, frequently lashing out at his parents and others who tried to help him. His rehabilitation was prolonged, punctuated by frequent bouts of sullen frustration. But slowly, almost imperceptibly, Will came to grips with his limitations.

Over the years, there were other changes as well. Will's parents, who had suffered doubt and sometimes despair during his aimless teens, discovered an inner strength that pulled them closer together than ever. His older brother, who had been more interested in following the Grateful Dead than in getting on with his life, gradually got his own act together and returned to college. His younger sister, mature beyond her years, became the confidante of her brothers.

And Dana, a beautiful young woman whose smile suggested a Latin *Mona Lisa*, just wouldn't go away. Despite Will's outbursts and the emotional roller coaster of his life, Dana slowly emerged as his most important constant, his pillar of strength. She was there when he learned each new task, not pushing him but, by her presence and enthusiasm, always encouraging him.

Together they re-entered college. Will needed taped lectures and a light load, but the stubbornness that had gotten him into trouble in his youth now began to pay dividends. His handicap became a challenge to be overcome, not a barrier to serve as an excuse. Last year, he and Dana graduated from college, and both hope to attend graduate school. And last week, in a college chapel in Pittsburgh, Dana and Will were married. The guests that filled the chapel were a blend of the cultures of the bride and groom. The ceremony itself was a celebration of love and determination, with tissues and handkerchiefs dabbing at eyes as each person recalled the events of the previous eight years.

Then, at the beginning of the recessional, Will, helped by Dana and a cane, got slowly and painfully to his feet. Sudden gasps were followed by applause and then free-flowing tears as he made his shuffling, one-step-at-a-time progress up the aisle. When he turned to his brother to help him get back into his wheelchair, and Dana kissed him and jumped into his lap, the applause turned to shouts of joy.

The story of Will and Dana no doubt will continue with its ups and downs. But if they make it through graduate school, have a family of their own, and have a long and fulfilling life together, I won't call it a miracle. Remember, I don't believe in miracles.

70

PAUSE BEFORE LABELING THIS MAN
HANDICAPPED

It's interesting to watch the way many of us treat people who have handicaps. Despite laws making overt discrimination illegal, we, nonetheless, too often discriminate in hundreds of small ways. For instance, we make assumptions about their preferences without asking them, we talk to them in condescending tones of voice, and we make decisions for them, as if they were children. And sometimes we even complain about them, as if their handicap is primarily an inconvenience for the rest of us.

An acquaintance of mine recently complained loudly when he saw a couple of vacant handicap parking spots in an otherwise crowded lot. I pointed out that opening up those two spots to everyone would have a trivial benefit for the able-bodied but it would come at a huge cost to the handicapped. He kept complaining.

Bill Weaver, the subject of a recent feature article in this newspaper, is severely handicapped. During the twenty-three years that I have known Bill, I have watched multiple sclerosis gradually change him from a strong, athletic man with infinite energy to a wheelchair-bound, easily fatigued individual who finds it difficult even to speak clearly when he is tired. But during the course of those twenty-three years, Bill's body was not the only thing that changed. For every physical skill Bill lost, he acquired new strengths in his determination to make a difference.

In addition to having a steady stream of great ideas, Bill has an incontrovertible ability to persuade others to work with him on projects. All his friends feel that stomach-turning mixture of excitement and dread when told, "Bill Weaver's on the phone for you." However, to those of his acquaintances who have watched his inexorable physical decline, Bill has been much more than an inspiration. He has been a teacher.

Maybe it's an innate human characteristic, but we seem to deal with people better when we can categorize them. Somehow, by labeling someone as white or black, or crippled, or gay, we begin to separate "them" from "us." The next step is to assume certain things about "them," and before long we feel comfortable in the knowledge that "we" are different from "them." Virtually all racial and homosexual stereotypes are based on just that logic. Bill Weaver and thousands like him teach us that the world just isn't that simple.

While it may be easy for us to categorize someone as crippled, Bill simply won't allow it. If asked to describe himself, my guess is that he would use a dozen or so labels—husband, father, businessman, community organizer, etc.—before it ever occurred to him to mention the word handicapped.

Jon Voight, in the powerful post-Vietnam war movie *Coming Home*, played a paraplegic Vietnam veteran. In one scene he talks of who he really is. He is not the paraplegic over there in a wheelchair. He is a complex man with fantasies, fears, ambition, love and, oh yes, a physical handicap.

We have come a long way, to be sure, from the days when handicapped people had no access to many of the things the rest of us take for granted. Despite its occasional abuses, the Americans with Disabilities Act has been a wonderful step forward in leveling the playing field. But just as civil rights legislation didn't change the way we think, the ADA is only the first step toward full participation by all of our citizens.

Our community has many problems, although far fewer than it would have if not for Bill Weaver. One step in addressing various issues is to develop talent whenever we find it. For those privileged to know him, perhaps Bill's greatest gift is that he has helped us examine those otherwise over-simplified categories, and see and fully appreciate the wonderfully complex and productive people behind the labels. As Dr. Seuss said in the voice of Horton the Elephant, "A person's a person no matter how small," from which we can extrapolate that a person's a person no matter WHAT!

71

IT'S A GOOD THING LAMAR DIDN'T LISTEN TO MY POLITICAL ADVICE

With Lamar Alexander's exit from the presidential race, I'm afraid my career as political consultant has also come to an end. But it was great while it lasted. Actually, Lamar, my friend of forty (gasp!) years, called on me for advice only on two occasions. Obviously he didn't want to bother me with the small things, like strategy for New Hampshire, or talking points on *Meet the Press*. No, he saved my ideas for really big political decisions.

The first was some time around January 1970. Lamar was working in the White House, and Carole and I were also living in the Washington area. We both had toddlers, and the four (or six) of us saw a lot of one another. One evening after dinner, Lamar sought my political wisdom for the first time. "I'm thinking of going back to Tennessee to help Winfield Dunn in his race for Governor. What do you think of that?"

"Lamar, that's the stupidest idea I've ever heard," I said, without a moment's hesitation. "You're on top of the world! Nixon will be re-elected, and a Republican dentist from Memphis doesn't have a chance to be governor of Tennessee."

The rest is history. Lamar left the White House, and by helping to get Dunn elected, he also began preparing himself for his own run for governor. Meanwhile, most of his associates from his White House days wound up disgraced, in jail, or both.

In those early years in politics, Lamar demonstrated traits that would make him a great governor. As far back as his college days, he had always been committed to doing things right. While ideology was important, Lamar had an instinct for what was doable. He saw that not only were good ideas important, but the ability to work with people, to compromise on some points in order to win others, and to maintain focus in the midst of all the background noise, were critical to success as a leader.

His start as governor in 1979 could not have been more inauspicious. Instead of the pomp and circumstance of a full-scale inauguration, Tennesseans suffered the embarrassment of watching their new governor being sworn in late one day in an emergency in order to curtail a major scandal in the outgoing administration. But that pained beginning didn't dampen his enthusiasm one bit, and he immediately went to work. The next eight years were a turning point in the history of our state.

Once again we had a governor of whom we could be proud. But most importantly, Tennessee gained visibility on the national scene. It's easy to take all of that for granted today, but try to think back on those days. Tennessee was pretty typical of the states of the Old South. With the exception of Georgia, we were all way behind the more industrialized states of the North and West. No one feels that way any more, and Lamar deserves a great deal of the credit for bringing Tennessee to where it is at the present.

Oh! I almost forgot. I said Lamar asked my advice not once, but twice. Again, he didn't want to waste my wisdom on little things like his Better Schools program, or the Saturn recruitment, or how to make contact with Japanese companies. He saved my counsel for bigger things.

It was the fall of 1977, and Lamar was gearing up for his second try at the governor's race, having lost in 1974 in the post-Watergate Democratic landslide. Once again, the four of us were out to dinner, and Lamar leaned over to me. "Tell you what I'm thinking about," he said. "I'm thinking of announcing my candidacy in Maryville in January, then walking all across the state, ending in Memphis on July Fourth. What do you think of that?"

"Lamar, that's the stupidest idea…"

72

HEALING HOLIDAY

My first Christmas as a physician was almost thirty years ago. I was an intern at the Johns Hopkins Hospital in Baltimore, and frankly, Christmas sneaked up on me that year. I knew it was late December, of course, and I had noticed the decorations, but I felt no real connection to their significance. Our intern schedule was the same as always—one night off each week—and Christmas was just another day. Or so it seemed.

Two or three days before Christmas itself, I was finishing up after a very long day and was heading home. In order to get there, I had to walk through the administration building, the oldest building in the Hopkins complex. As I walked down the corridor, I was startled by some of the sweetest music I had ever heard—the sounds of a local, all-black church choir rehearsing in preparation to tour the hospital and serenade the patients. There were few dry eyes in the group of doctors and nurses who had interrupted their routines to share in the moment.

And it's been the same ever since. Whether in Baltimore, Bethesda, New York, or Nashville, hospitals are special places at this time of year. Whether Christian or not—indeed, whether religious or not —this season is a special time when we pause and realize that, after all is said and done, individual acts of kindness and love are what this season is all about.

Maybe this is the best time of year to be a physician, nurse, or other caregiver. We see people like Vanessa, a single mother on TennCare, who has maintained her spirit despite a disfiguring and debilitating disease, and who took the time and made the effort to bring a tray of cheese and sausages to our clinic doctors and nurses.

There was Tom, the patient who was so enthusiastic in his attempt to give us a country ham that he walked right into an examination room. He didn't mind, and by the way, neither did the patient. Years after his death, we still talk of Tom's joy in sharing.

And there's Regina, whose rheumatoid arthritis has progressively crippled her but hasn't dampened her enthusiasm for preparing a wonderful batch of candy for our clinic staff year after year. Likewise, Carole, whose illness leaves her in constant pain, can't wait to share her prized apple-nut bread.

There's also Joy and her fellow nurses, whose Christmas party for their patients has turned into a day-long celebration of love and friendship. And Yarrot and his late brother, Charlie, who dropped by on Christmas Eve many years ago with a gift I shall treasure forever.

Medicine is a strange profession. While the highs are truly incredible, the fact is that much of a doctor or nurse's day is spent doing routine, rather mundane work. But then there is this wonderful time of year when people give of themselves in ways even they could not have predicted. The outpouring of love and willingness to share and help one another are especially visible around hospitals and clinics, and it is always these times when those of us in medicine know that this is about as good as it can get.

If someone ever asks me the true meaning of Christmas, I will tell them about a very tired intern on a late December night in Baltimore about thirty years ago.

73

AN ORTHODOX CHRISTMAS

Christmas 1991 was approaching, but we were looking forward to it with mixed feelings. We were excited about having Katie home from college and Ellen home from Washington, where she had moved after graduation, but as Christmas drew nearer, the anxiety and tension increased daily.

It had been nearly two years since my father's death, and that fact weighed heavily on the holiday. We knew we would find constant reminders of his ever-present smile and gentle demeanor, but the reason for the tension was the stress of dealing with my mother's continuing grief. His death had caused her to sink into a shell of despair and loneliness that we were powerless to dent, and her sadness often became contagious, especially during holidays. On Christmas Eve morning we had a big breakfast and tried to involve my mother in our activities, but she had little interest in anything we suggested.

Then the phone rang, and it was Katie's friend from school who was traveling around the South with four of his friends. Knowing that he was an Orthodox Jew, Katie asked if he needed help finding kosher food, but he assured her that they had plenty of kosher peanut butter, cheese, and cereal, and that they were doing fine. The day was cold and dreary, and as Katie was getting ready to drive out to their campground, Carole and I simultaneously insisted that she invite them over. All of our bedrooms were occupied, but we had plenty of couch and floor space.

As soon as they drove up we knew we were in for a treat. Bouncing out of their van were five well-mannered young men with South African accents, obviously delighted at the prospect of spending the night in a warm home instead of a campground. They had been childhood friends, and four were attending various colleges in the United States. The fifth was visiting from Johannesburg. As soon as they saw the Christmas tree and all of our decorations, it became clear they had never spent Christmas in a Christian home, and they wanted to know the significance of everything.

We showed them every ornament on the tree, and as we did, each decoration took on special significance for us as well. We told stories of ornaments Carole had made from Styrofoam when we were first married, ornaments celebrating the births of our children and places we had lived, and symbols representing relatives and special friendships. We explained everything, from the history of the stockings hung on the mantle to the crèche scenes, and they told us their own stories of celebrations on special occasions. After getting over her bewilderment at the whole scene, my mother chimed in, obviously enjoying reliving the history of our family.

Christmas morning found our living room covered with sleeping bags. After serving as traffic engineers to cycle our visitors and family through the showers, we went about the task of preparing Christmas dinner. Our guests insisted on eating their cheese and peanut butter, but we were pretty sure we could come up with something better. A quick phone call to our neighbors, also Orthodox Jews, revealed that they maintained a supply of frozen kosher meals for just such occasions. So our Christmas table that year was filled with our family eating turkey and all the trimmings, and five young men eating Cornish game hens on plastic plates. The prayer before the meal, calling for love and understanding, never seemed more appropriate.

Until her death six years later, my mother never really got over the loss of my father. I'm not sure she even wanted to. We tried our best year after year, but she seemed to have decided that with his death, happiness wasn't any longer something to which she could aspire. So Christmas in particular, was always difficult for us during those years...always, that is, except for that one special year when five young Jews helped us appreciate the joys and traditions of this wonderful season.

74

SAVE TIME AT CHRISTMAS
TO TELL ABOUT THOSE GONE

My friend and former teacher, Dr. Charles Wells, writes Christmas stories. They aren't the "See how great my life is. Isn't it a shame yours is so ordinary?" letters that make me want to reach for the Dramamine, and they aren't stories of Christmas, really. What Charles does is write a several-page story about someone or something that matters to him. This year's was the story of Clyde, a boyhood friend who had recently died and whose good humor made Charles' life at military school almost bearable.

When my father died fifteen years ago, I experienced a sense of loss that I had not anticipated. He had been ill for several months and I thought I had prepared myself for the inevitable. However, what I wasn't prepared for was the sudden realization that not only was he gone, but that our common story was in danger of being lost as well. No longer could I call him to celebrate a sports event, or to ask about some long-departed relative, or just to say hello. I sensed in Charles' story of Clyde some of that same longing, the feeling that Clyde's physical demise should not be the end of his story.

For Christians, this is the time of the year when we often stop to call or write someone just to say how much they mean to us. We hear a great deal these days about putting meaning back into Christmas and unfortunately, most of it is a lot of nonsense. It is hard to imagine that anyone, much less God, cares how we greet people in this season. Instead, many of us who think about the meaning of Christmas, recall times long ago, when Christmas meant the wonder and mystery of childhood. Santa Claus was part of it for a few years of course, but primarily we hearken back to the innocence of youth, which offered the belief that those around us were always going to be there, and that the world was a safe and inviting place.

As we age, that innocence is replaced by the realization that illness and death are a part of life, and we have to choose how we will deal with it. For many, the sad events of life gradually turn them into depressed and lonely people. Others find great solace in religion, and in many cases experience meaning and spiritual growth even in the face of sadness. Still others find comfort in simply telling the stories of those they love. One longtime friend, Sigourney Cheek, is taking time out from her own battle with cancer to write her story, which is intertwined with the important role her father played in her life.

When one of my daughters was in grade school her teacher asked her to tape an oral history of an older person. She went across the street to visit Henry Goodpasture. Then in his eighties and still practicing law, Henry told Ellen wonderful tales of his childhood and his friends and associates from long ago. As she was leaving, he handed her a manuscript he had prepared years before. It was dedicated to his sons, Ken, a minister and theologian, and Jim, who had been brain-injured at birth and lived in an institution elsewhere. Jim came to stay with Henry and Virginia several times a year, and he enjoyed walking tirelessly up and down the street, picking up bits of paper and other trash. In the dedication at the beginning of his manuscript, Henry wrote that they both had taught him, in different ways, the meaning of love. The manuscript covered Henry's life story, and it was so interesting I told him he should publish it. His reply was straightforward and typical. "I didn't write it to be published, John. I wrote it for myself."

Tomorrow I will pause once more not only to remember those who will never again spend Christmas with me, but also to remember the thrill of falling in love with Carole, the exhilaration of the births of Ellen and Katie, and the heart-bursting joy that our grandchildren have brought. And I'll tell each one just how much they mean to me. After all, they are inseparable parts of my story, just as I am of theirs.

75

CHRISTMAS TREE

Last week for the thirty-ninth time, Carole and I decorated our Christmas tree. It's always special, with the smell of the tree somehow canceling the knowledge that by the time Christmas is over, we will be all too happy to lug it down to the recycling pick-up area and get our house back to normal.

Christmas trees are one of a number of pagan practices that were long ago adopted by Christianity. In what is now Germany and in other parts of Europe, the practice of celebrating the winter solstice by brightening up the house with greenery was commonplace. When those areas became Christianized, this tradition was adopted by the new religion. And although the religious connotations of Christmas are worth celebrating, days getting longer and spring getting closer are also worth celebrating in their own right.

So, following our pagan and then our Christian ancestors, Carole and I strung the lights on the tree, put an angel on top, and then began adding the ornaments. One by one we pulled them out, pausing to remember the story behind each. Most of our oldest ones were handmade, for reasons both personal and financial. We paused with every one, thinking of friends, some from as far back as my internship year, who we now remember only with annual Christmas cards.

There were ornaments given to us by friends and relatives who have died, and each of those received special handling. There were ornaments representing weddings, births of grandchildren, and special vacations. When we finished, our tree was a splish-splash of colors and decorations, but we decided it was perfect, although looking at all of those ornaments suddenly made us realize how much we've aged in nearly forty years of marriage.

The process of aging is so gradual that we almost don't notice it. I know the connective tissues around my joints get a little bit stiffer every day, my maximum attainable heart rate declines in a straight-line fashion year by year, and my ability to exercise and consume oxygen falls a tiny amount daily, and I know I can't prevent any of it. If you don't believe it, check the world records by age group for the mile run or the marathon.

So we merrily go along, skin sagging and hair graying by such a miniscule bit more each day that we don't think of aging much at all. Then we do something like trim a Christmas tree, and all those memories come flooding in. For a while the act of recalling seems almost more than we can stand—the dear friends, our wonderful grandchildren, the Christmases when we couldn't afford it but bought a tree just the same. With all of those thoughts, the fact that we have aged is suddenly undeniable. Full of nostalgia, we think for a moment about how much we would like to have those years—and those friends and relatives—with us again.

That can't happen, of course, and soon we get over our wishing and yearning. Before we know it we are getting out the toys for grandson Henry to play with when he will come the next day, to be joined soon after by his cousins Kathryn and Emmaline. In this joyous anticipation our "maturing" doesn't seem so bad after all, less a curse than a blessing. We are at peace. Merry Christmas.

76

CAPTIVATING SWEETHEART
TAKES DOCTOR AS PRISONER

There's another woman in my life. After thirty-seven years of marriage and two grown daughters, I love someone else in ways I never dreamed would be possible. I think about her all day, I dream of her at night, and I find myself window shopping for any little thing that might please her.

The thing that amazes me most is that despite my feelings for her, she couldn't care less whether I'm around or not. And when I am with her, she glances right past me as if I didn't even exist. But I don't care. Her every gesture, every facial expression, is burned in my memory. Her face is the last thing I visualize before falling asleep, and it's my first thought every morning. When we are apart, I wonder what she's doing and how she will look when I next see her.

I never thought it would be this way for me. I've watched other men in similar situations and listened to them describe their love and joy, and thought it just wouldn't happen to me. I figured these were people who had simply gone a little bit crazy in their advancing years. And then I met Kathryn, and was immediately transformed into a blubbering idiot, not only willing, but anxious to tell the world of my bursting love.

Kathryn is my brand new granddaughter, and she is beautiful. She seems to have her mother's mouth and her father's eyes, but I'm not very skilled at picking up resemblances; mostly she looks like a baby. Maybe that's part of what makes her so special. She lies there, eyes trying to focus, helpless except for the ability to cry when hungry, and yet within her is the potential to be anything: senator, ballerina, athlete, actress, mother, scientist.

Added to my joy over her birth is the surprise and pride I feel in watching my own child in a new role. How can it be that Ellen, whose diaper I've changed, whose tears I've dried, whose cuts and scrapes I've treated, can be so competent and comfortable in her newest and most important job yet, that of being a parent? But there she is just the same, confident enough to point out to her mother and me that the baby bed so lovingly kept all these years, the bed that nurtured her and her sister, didn't meet modern standards and would have to be replaced.

It's the same with Kathryn's father, Jon, an outstanding young man whose love for Ellen immediately put him on a pedestal in my heart. Jon is skilled in many things, but watching him hold his daughter with that look of total devotion elevated him to a new level. Kathryn is a very lucky little girl.

Something else makes her really special. When Carole and I became parents, we were still very young ourselves. We enjoyed our children immensely, but our lives were hectic and our future uncertain. Now we are approaching the end of our careers and are much more aware of our own mortality. In a very tangible sense, Kathryn reminds us that some part of us will still be here after we're gone.

So, overcome with love, I look into unfocused eyes that may one day capture the heart of some young man, I look at those tiny fingers that in the years to come may hold her own child, and I think of the joy and even the occasional heartache she will bring to her parents.

Whatever her future holds, one thing is certain: my life will never be the same.

77

IT CAN BE A RUSH FOR INFORMATION
WHEN A CHILD'S HEALTH SEEMS FISHY

Kathryn, our five-year-old granddaughter, loved school from day one…all but the fish lunches and the chicken costume, but we'll get to that. She loved her new friends, her teachers, and her art projects, and she especially loved learning to read. I had forgotten just how thrilling it is to watch a child begin the process of putting letters together to form sounds and then whole words. Although she was pretty tired at the end of each day, Kathryn would jump out of bed the next morning, excited and looking forward to the day.

As to the fish, her school serves a really nutritious lunch every day. No junk food. At least once a week they serve fish, usually something like baked cod or broiled trout. Kathryn doesn't like fish and invariably comes home hungry on fish day. Fish for lunch, and the fact that for the school play her class had to wear chicken costumes, were the only unenthusiastic things Kathryn had to say about her school.

Then a few weeks ago, things began to change. She seemed more fatigued at the end of the day, and her enthusiasm for school in the mornings had waned. She no longer worked endlessly on art projects, and she became fussy, sometimes arguing with her little sister and her friends. Her parents began to worry that something was wrong, but they didn't have much to go on until they noticed small ridges forming across some of her fingernails. They took her straight to the doctor.

Their physician noted that Kathryn had not gained any weight in six months and he drew blood for some tests. After an anxious several hours we were told that the routine studies looked okay, which was a relief, but that still left us wondering what was wrong. The following day he told us that Kathryn had blood test results compatible with celiac disease, and that she should undergo a biopsy of her small intestine to confirm the diagnosis.

When I was in medical school, celiac disease was thought to be an extremely rare condition that usually caused severe diarrhea and wasting. Now we know that it is fairly common, with nearly one percent of the population afflicted, according to some surveys, and overt gastrointestinal symptoms, the most common indicator, are not necessarily present at all. The disease is a complex one in which genetic and environmental factors interact to damage the small intestine. The people affected with the disease develop an immune reaction to gluten, a substance found in wheat, rye, and barley. That reaction injures the cells of the intestinal lining, resulting in failure to absorb nutrients needed for growth. Treatment is lifelong complete elimination of gluten from the diet, something made more difficult by the fact that gluten is often added for its thickening and binding effects to a variety of foods, even things like ice cream.

Upon hearing this probable diagnosis, Kathryn's mother Ellen immediately got online. You haven't seen anyone attack the Internet until you see a concerned mother trying to learn all she can about something she had only first heard of a few days before. Hour after hour Ellen took notes on potato and rice flour, acceptable ice cream brands, Internet food delivery services, gluten-free cookbooks, and much more. Even before the diagnosis was confirmed, she began teaching Kathryn that she may be allergic to wheat and what that might mean, such as not eating the cake at birthday parties, having her own special pizza, and so on.

Thanks to fiberoptic technology, the biopsy itself wasn't a big deal; however, in children it requires general anesthesia. The doctor met with us immediately afterwards and showed us pictures of Kathryn's intestinal lining (that she would later describe as "Yucky"), and said he was virtually certain the biopsies would show celiac disease, which turned out to be the case.

As Kathryn was waking from the anesthesia and getting her bearings, she asked, "Mommy, what did the doctor find when he looked in my tummy?" "He found that you are allergic to wheat, Honey. That means you can't eat things that have wheat in them," Ellen replied.

Kathryn thought about that for a minute, and then said, "Mommy, does fish have wheat in it?"

78

BOBBY KENNEDY'S DEATH REMEMBERED

Last week's 40th anniversary of the death of Bobby Kennedy brought back a surge of memories and emotions. We were living in Baltimore, the proud parents of three-month-old Ellen, but it was an extremely troubling time. Over the previous two years, race riots had already occurred in a number of U.S. cities, and to make matters worse, we were bogged down in the divisive and seemingly endless war in Vietnam.

On April 4, 1968, when Ellen was not yet one month old, Martin Luther King, Jr., was killed. There were riots all over the country, none worse than in Baltimore. We felt relatively safe thanks to the widespread deployment of the Maryland National Guard, but the appearance of the city engulfed in hundreds of fires looked as if we were being bombed. On the Sunday after King's death, Carole and Ellen went to stay with friends in a safe area of Washington. I told them goodbye, uncertain how long it would be before we would be together again, and went to the hospital with the air still thick with smoke.

Over the next few days, things gradually quieted down, and after a week or so our family was reunited, but Baltimore remained tense. The anxiety was noticeable even at the hospital, where black nurses I had worked with on a daily basis seemed guarded and suspicious, and maybe they felt that way about me. Regardless, the normally friendly banter among doctors and nurses was replaced by more formal interactions that were strange and unfamiliar. We were all on guard, certain that the slightest slip of the tongue would be construed the wrong way.

Two months after King's death, Bobby Kennedy was killed. When he had spoken of visiting the Mississippi Delta and seeing the poverty and suffering there, and of coming away determined to do something about it, he struck a chord among many, especially African-Americans. His nomination seemed assured the night he won the California primary and then, as the nation watched, he was shot and it was over. Coming less than five years after his brother's assassination and only two months after King's, it was a low point for the country, and especially for African-Americans.

On the Sunday after Bobby Kennedy's death, I suggested to Carole that we try to cheer up and take a little ride, maybe go to a park and take Ellen for a walk. As we began to drive through East Baltimore, we noticed groups of well-dressed black people walking along the streets. The first groups we saw were small, but as we drove farther the crowds swelled, sometimes several dozen strong, all walking silently. Some had tears streaming down their faces. There were old people with canes and young people carrying babies. As we came to a railroad overpass, we suddenly realized what was happening. The train carrying Kennedy's body from New York to his burial at Arlington was coming through Baltimore, and people were turning out by the thousands to pay their respects. They lined the tracks all along the large swath the train cut through the city, silently honoring their fallen hero.

The next day I told one of the African-American nurses what I had seen, and she proudly told me that she and her family were there. For the first time, we openly shared our emotions and sense of loss. In a city still sharply divided by race, we realized that we shared something much more important: we were Americans, and we were suffering, but we were starting to heal.

79

TEE TIME

Middle-aged. It automatically conjures up related phrases such as receding hairline, flabby arms, enlarged prostate, and a variety of orthopaedic ailments.

When you stop to think about it, *middle age* is a peculiar term. The implication is that a middle-aged person is halfway through life, but I don't know any 106-year-old people, so it must mean something else. Maybe it's the expanding waistline most of us develop that gives this period of life its name. At any rate, as a group, we are larger in the middle, so the term fits pretty well.

And do we fight it! We take vitamins, go to health spas, try exotic diets, undergo hair transplants, get facelifts and adjustments to assorted other areas, and generally try our best to avoid looking— or acting—our age. The results of all this are frequently humorous and occasionally disastrous, as in the case of a friend who tore up his shoulder and nearly killed himself while buzzing around on a moped. I'm talking about someone who hasn't been on as much as a bicycle in years, but there he was, on vacation, unable to resist the urge to relive a youthful experience he probably never had in the first place.

Then there's the plastic surgery that has become a ritual these days, much as our children had to pass through orthodontics on their way to their teens. There is almost no limit to the pain and discomfort we middle-agers will put ourselves through to look younger. It is perhaps a fitting testimonial to our era that when

Audrey Hepburn died, she was eulogized in *The New York Times* for, among other things, not having had a facelift.

This year, at last, I had to face reality. The hills at Percy Warner Park had gotten steeper every year, and my surgically repaired shoulder sent me painful reminders of my age after each tennis match. Increasingly, getting out of bed after an active weekend had become a stiff process requiring some planning. And those extra pounds picked up on vacation just wouldn't go away.

Yes, I must have entered middle age. To mark the occasion, I decided to take up the quintessential middle-ager's game. I took a golf lesson. It wasn't easy taking up golf. I had always felt so superior to the golfers at Percy Warner Park as I ran up the hills. I had snickered when friends took trips just to play golf, while I packed tennis racquets and running shoes. And when my cousin and his wife, who used to battle tooth-and-nail with us in tennis on 100-degree days, called last year to say they had started playing golf, my only comment was, "I'll never be that old!"

So I had to eat a little crow when I showed up for my lesson wearing tennis shoes alongside all those well-shined oxfords with their confident, clicking sounds as they strolled along the sidewalk. And then I made a shocking discovery: golf is harder than it looks.

But my twenty-something-year-old daughters came through. For my birthday, they wanted to give me an appropriate gift for my new activity. I expected maybe a new putter, or a three wood, but they gave me something I really needed: a ball retriever for fishing balls out of the water. And, comfortably in middle age as I am, I didn't even mind.

80

ANOTHER YEAR OLDER
AND MORE BLESSINGS THAN EVER

Birthdays have never mattered much to me. Maybe it's because genetics and luck have combined to keep me healthy, so I don't feel much older than I did ten or even twenty years ago. Two weeks ago, though, I turned sixty, and while taking my annual birthday run, I have to say it got to me a little.

First of all, there was the pace of the run itself. A longtime friend was running alongside me one morning a couple of months ago, and she commented that a few years ago we would have called what we were doing jogging, or trotting, or even fast walking, but not running!

Then there's the whole "middle-aged" thing. I'm not psychologically ready to be called a senior citizen, but there aren't many 120-year-olds around. Fortunately, any negative connotations associated with turning sixty were softened by the circumstances. We were on vacation at the beach with both of our children and their families, which included two-month-old Henry and sixteen-month-old Kathryn. Henry, Katie and Dave's son, has cheeks that make the Gerber baby look underfed, and intermittently he has a huge, lopsided, gaping smile that would totally melt my heart if I didn't know he was focusing on the ceiling fan instead of his grandfather.

Kathryn, Ellen and Jon's daughter, was simultaneously getting over an ear infection and cutting four teeth, and therefore required more than the usual amount of holding and comforting, which her grandmother and I were only too happy to provide. As I took her on bike rides and played with her in the sand, I couldn't help but remember my children at that age, and, probably stimulated by my birthday, I thought a lot about my father, who had died thirteen years ago.

My father had a beautiful tenor voice, a trait I didn't inherit, and every night until I was twelve or thirteen, we sang songs at bedtime. We sang everything from "Stardust" and other songs of the '30s and '40s, to hymns and mountain spirituals, to college songs. To this day I know all the words to "Let's Drink a Toast to Dear Old Maine" despite never to my knowledge knowing a single person who actually went to college there. My favorites, though, were two sailing songs. One was "Sailing, Sailing, Over the Bounding Main," and the other was "A Capital Ship for an Ocean Trip," about a boy with a vivid imagination who converts his bed into a ship.

Despite my inability to carry a tune, I continued the tradition with my children, standing in the middle of their room and teaching five-year-old Ellen to pause so her sister could chime in with the few words she knew. During our vacation, Ellen and I tried to get Kathryn to sing, but with a vocabulary of only about thirty words, it's hard to construct much of a song, especially when a good percentage of her vocabulary is devoted to body parts, including "belly button," a term I don't believe has ever been put to music.

I didn't accomplish everything I had planned on that vacation. I only got part way through David McCullough's biography of John Adams, for example. But in many ways it couldn't have been better. I saw my children happily married and becoming wonderful mothers. I saw a side of my wife Carole as grandmother that I never expected: She actually let her granddaughter play ball in the house. I listened to Kathryn count to three, figuring that with such math skills the only question in 2019 will be whether she goes to Cal Tech or MIT.

I came home realizing once again that aging, and even death itself, can't stop some things. In our family, one of those is bedtime singing. Incidentally, we also celebrated Father's Day while we were away. Thanks again, Daddy.

81

HAPPINESS

Commencement is a time for looking forward, but it is also a time for reflection. As I watched the brand new doctors receive their degrees from Vanderbilt last week, I couldn't help but reflect on my class over forty years ago and what became of us. Just like this year's graduates, we were full of optimism and enthusiasm as we embarked on our careers, but the years have not treated us all the same. Some of us have had rich, happy lives and others have not.

In Jonathon Haidt's excellent book, *The Happiness Hypothesis*, he explores the various factors that make an individual happy. First, according to Haidt, there is genetic predisposition—some of us innately see the world in a positive, optimistic light while others do not. Those who are innately happy, according to Haidt, have won what he refers to as the "cortical lottery."

He goes on, though, to examine other characteristics of happy people, and he points out that the usual things we strive for, especially wealth, are not strongly associated with happiness. Indeed, once basic needs are taken care of, there is little correlation at all between wealth and happiness. So what kinds of people tend to be happiest? As you might expect, they are people with deep friendships, usually many of them, and part of being a friend is developing relationships based on mutual trust and sharing.

If you think of the worst thing that could happen to you—going blind, being paralyzed, losing a spouse or child—your first thought might be that you could not live with such a tragedy, yet we all know people who do, in fact, live rich, full lives despite overwhelming disability or personal loss. Nashville businessman Bill Weaver, who died of multiple sclerosis last December, was just such a person. Despite many years of quadriplegia, he maintained a wide circle of friends, loved conversation, and kept his terrific sense of humor right up to his death.

My friend Melvin Fitzgerald is another model of a happy man. For fifty-one years Melvin has worked as an office assistant in the Department of Biochemistry at Vanderbilt. He seems to know everyone in the medical center, and in 1996 he received the Commodore Award, the highest award for a member of the Vanderbilt staff. When Melvin's wife of over twenty-five years, Trinita, died a couple of years ago, he was visibly saddened for months, but slowly his warmth and friendliness returned. While life will never be the same, he continues to nurture a large circle of friends including people at work, members of his church, and a group of men he has breakfast with every Saturday. While Melvin undoubtedly won the cortical lottery, he has also gone out of his way to develop relationships that matter, and those relationships have sustained him.

Dr. Bob Fisher, president of Belmont University, and his wife Judy have written a book based on interviews with people in Alive Hospice. In their book, *Life Is a Gift: Inspiration From the Soon Departed*, they ask dying people what their message is for the rest of us. None spoke of accumulating wealth or possessions; instead, virtually all of them spoke of the importance of relationships. Not surprisingly, the Fishers point out time and again in their book that those people with strong relationships almost always faced their deaths with few or no regrets. And when you think about it, dying with no regrets is almost certainly the best measure of a life well lived.

More information on the Fishers' book is available at:
www.alivehospice.org

APPENDIX

*All articles are published by permission and originally appeared
in the Nashville* Tennessean.

AUTHOR BIOGRAPHY

John Sergent was born in West Virginia and grew up in Kentucky. He graduated from Vanderbilt University with a BA degree in 1963 and from Vanderbilt University Medical School in 1966. He completed his graduate training in internal medicine and rheumatology at Johns Hopkins, the National Institutes of Health, Vanderbilt, and Cornell. In addition to nine years in private practice, he has spent the remainder of his career on the Vanderbilt faculty. He was the university's first chief of rheumatology, then later served as Chief of Medicine at St. Thomas Hospital and subsequently was the first Chief Medical Officer of the Vanderbilt Medical Group. He currently serves as vice chair for education of the Department of Medicine and is the director of the internal medicine residency program.

His greatest love is teaching, for which he has received numerous awards from his peers as well as his students. In 2007 Vanderbilt established an annual teaching award in his name.

He was President of the American College of Rheumatology and has been selected as a Master in both the American College of Rheumatology and the American College of Physicians. He is a co-editor of the leading textbook in rheumatology. For over fifteen years he has been a regular op-ed columnist for the Nashville *Tennessean*, from which these essays were collected.

Dr. Sergent is married and has two daughters. His greatest current pleasure is spoiling his four grandchildren.